Clinical Skills in Psychiatric Treatment

Clinical Skills in Psychiatric Treatment

ROB POOLE AND ROBERT HIGGO

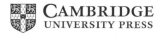
CAMBRIDGE
UNIVERSITY PRESS

CAMBRIDGE UNIVERSITY PRESS
Cambridge, New York, Melbourne, Madrid, Cape Town, Singapore, São Paulo, Delhi

Cambridge University Press
The Edinburgh Building, Cambridge CB2 8RU, UK

Published in the United States of America by Cambridge University Press, New York

www.cambridge.org
Information on this title: www.cambridge.org/9780521705707

First published 2008

Printed in the United Kingdom at the University Press, Cambridge

A catalogue record for this publication is available from the British Library

Library of Congress Cataloguing in Publication Data

Poole, Rob, 1956–
Clinical skills in psychiatric treatment / Rob Poole and Robert Higgo.
    p. ; cm. – (Cambridge clinical guides)
Includes bibliographical references and index.
ISBN- 978-0-521-70570-7 (pbk.)
1. Mental illness – Treatment – Standards.   2. Psychiatry – Standards.   3. Clinical competence.
I. Higgo, Robert, 1952–   II. Title.   III. Series.
[DNLM: 1. Clinical Competence.   2. Mental Disorders – therapy.   WM 21 P822c 2008]
RC480.5.P634   2008
616.89′1–dc22   20070521269

ISBN 978-0-521-70570-7 hardback

This book is dedicated to the late Leo Fender, whose supreme mastery of the art of guitar design was unencumbered by an ability to play the instrument.

Contents

Acknowledgments	*page* ix
Author biographies	xi
Introduction	1

PART I – UNDERLYING PRINCIPLES

1 Starting points	7
2 A triangle of forces	13
3 Treatment objectives	21
4 Strategic treatment	30

PART II – THE CONTEXT AND LOCATION OF TREATMENT

5 Teams	45
6 Teamwork	56
7 Inpatient treatment in the era of community psychiatry	68
8 Compulsion and locked doors	81
9 Not at home, not in hospital	88
10 Models of care	97

PART III – PROBLEMS IN TREATMENT

11 Engagement	111
12 Compliance and concordance	121
13 Treatment resistance	134
14 Complicated problems	149
15 Managing risk	161
16 Staying well	176

PART IV – COPING

17 Coping with dilemmas   191

18 Coping with change   203

Afterword: Optimism of the will and pessimism of the intellect   213

References   217

Index   221

Acknowledgments

The idea for this book came to us on the day that we returned the corrected proofs of our last book to the publisher. That book had taken almost a decade to write, and we realised that we had to change our modus operandi. Ponderous debate gave way to reckless hastiness, and this book has been less than two years in preparation. If we have managed to produce a worthwhile text, it is in large measure due to the selfless support of family, friends and colleagues.

Draft material was read by Vinnie Farrell, Gordon Kennedy, Julie Kenny, Theresa McArdle, Prem Muthuvelu, Chris Quinn, Paul Rowlands, Jenny Smith, Gill Strong and Kate Wood. We are grateful for their thoughtful comments, which have improved the text considerably.

We must especially thank Sue Ruben, who read draft material, loaned us her cottage so that we could write without distraction, and painted the cover illustration. We also thank Steve Hammond for providing photographic services at short notice.

Our employers have generously supported the project through provision of study leave. We are particularly grateful to our medical managers, Giles Harbourne and David Fearnley, in this regard.

We seem to have developed a distinctive style of writing that creates books about psychiatry that are a little unconventional. We must thank Richard Marley of Cambridge University Press for his unstinting encouragement to produce books that say what we want to say in the way that we want to say it.

Finally, we must thank Greta, Geoff, Audrey and Arthur, who made all of this possible.

Author biographies

Rob Poole

Rob Poole grew up in South East London. He is a general adult psychiatrist with a strong interest in the psychological, social and cultural aspects of mental illness. After training at St George's Hospital, London and in Oxford, he worked for many years as a consultant psychiatrist in a deprived part of Liverpool, before moving to his current post in rural North Wales. He has extensive experience of leading service development and of establishing new models of team working. He has a strong background in teaching and postgraduate education, and he has dabbled in research.

Robert Higgo

Robert Higgo grew up in Cape Town. He had experience of working in general practice and public health medicine prior to training in psychiatry in Liverpool. This has helped to shape his psychosocial approach to psychiatric practice. He has worked as a general adult psychiatrist in Merseyside and Manchester, and he is presently the consultant psychiatrist for the Liverpool Assertive Outreach Team. His main interests have been in postgraduate medical education and training at all levels, and in reviewing adverse incidents in clinical practice both locally and nationally. He is an enthusiastic supporter of New Ways of Working for Psychiatrists.

Introduction

This book is concerned with treatment strategies that facilitate recovery from mental illness. We have attempted to outline ideas and ways of thinking that assist in the development of clinical skills and the effective use of treatment technologies in the real world. This is not a primer on psychopharmacology, nor a guide to specific psychological or social therapies. Indeed, it is assumed that readers have some basic knowledge of these subjects. Instead, we explore the application of principles to everyday work, and the ways around the numerous complications, pitfalls and dilemmas that are the stuff of clinical practice.

In many ways, making treatments work for patients in the face of the complications and problems of real life is the most difficult aspect of the work of mental health professionals. It demands a good understanding of scientific evidence, combined with an empathic understanding of other people and an ability to constructively learn from clinical experience. Above all, clinicians have to be self-aware and conscious that treatment can do harm as well as good. At its heart, this book is about the difference between comprehensive knowledge and good clinical skills.

This text follows on from our previous work, *Psychiatric Interviewing and Assessment*, which was concerned with fundamental skills that lead to good quality assessment and facilitate a therapeutic relationship. However, although it is informed by the same values, this volume stands on its own. It aims to help clinicians to develop the ability to work with patients to create rational and strategic treatment plans, so that the overall intervention is user friendly and constructive. It is based on an understanding of the complexities and problems that arise in everyday practice, where the planning and implementation of treatment has to take account of a multitude of contextual factors and unexpected events.

As a consequence of our attempts to give the material a 'real life' quality, the text bears the clear imprint of our experience as practising psychiatrists. We have primarily addressed the book to psychiatrists in the UK who, having acquired the necessary technical knowledge, are dealing with the problems of autonomous clinical practice. However, we believe that the concepts herein have relevance to a wide group of clinicians, including mental health nurses, social workers, psychologists and occupational therapists. We also believe that very little in the book is unique to British practice, and we hope that it will be useful to clinicians in other countries. In order to reach a broad readership, we have tried to balance the authenticity that comes from writing from personal experience with a generalised approach to allow applicability across disciplines and countries. We should acknowledge, however, that this book will be useful mainly to mental health professionals who treat mental illness in people of working age.

There are numerous fictional clinical vignettes in the text. We have taken care to make these realistic, but they are not based on any individual patient's history or presentation. Where a story is true, we have said so. All of the others have been invented, albeit on the basis of situations that really do happen.

We have followed some conventions that might appear to be slightly at odds with our commitment to patient orientated, non-discriminatory, evidence-based practice. We have sometimes used the term 'patient' rather than 'service user'. We do not believe that the concept of the doctor–patient relationship is outmoded, and we set out one good reason for this in Chapter 17. We have used male pronouns generically, because, being men, we find it easier to write that way. We apologise to female colleagues for this. We have made some compromises in order to maintain readability. In particular, we have limited the number of references, mainly using them to direct readers towards important publications, or to provide evidence for points that might be contentious. We have avoided referencing well-recognised and widely accepted facts and concepts. We have expressed some very firm opinions, some of which may be controversial. This is not an attempt to press our idiosyncratic views on others. We believe that such opinions are inevitable, and we have tried to explain how our opinions have been formed, in order to illustrate the problem of balancing evidence, beliefs, values and rationality. We fully recognise that some of our dearly held opinions will eventually prove to be wrong.

In the past, it often seemed that the multidisciplinary team was a group of professionals with different ways of understanding mental disorder, who followed (or sometimes subverted) plans under the direction of a consultant psychiatrist. Lately British psychiatrists have been encouraged to adopt new ways of working, which really means fully embracing proper multidisciplinary teamwork. Modern teams are a group of professionals sharing a common, multifaceted understanding, who bring their different skills to a jointly owned plan. We both work in teams whose practices reflect the new patterns of work, and the book is strongly informed by this experience. However, we have also tried to address issues that arise in smaller teams or in the course of single-handed working.

In places, we have dwelt at length upon issues of control of patients and of the use of medication. We fully recognise that recovery can only be the result of treatment when clinicians get alongside patients rather than controlling them. We also recognise that medication is often a regrettable necessity. Interventions are likely to fail if medication is the predominant element. There are many problems associated with psychotropic medication, but it cannot be eliminated from clinical practice, and for this reason it has to receive some emphasis. However, the central tactic in most treatment strategies is stepwise problem solving, not medication.

We have written this book in the hope that it will be read rather than consulted. We do not suppose that we are exceptionally able clinicians who can put colleagues right through a didactic exposition of our ideas. To the best of our knowledge, the concepts set out here have not been the subject of a book before, but they are well known to many experienced clinicians of all disciplines. They are formed from experience, from discovering what works and what does not, and from what our patients tell us. We hope to help readers to develop skills. We have aimed to provoke rather than to inform, in the belief that the best teaching is thought provoking and entertaining.

Part I – Underlying principles

These first four chapters set out the underlying principles of rational, strategic treatment. Chapter 1 deals with some important values and reiterates some themes from our previous book. Chapter 2 is concerned with balancing contextual factors, scientific evidence and clinical experience to produce treatments that are rational and appropriate. Chapter 3 emphasises the importance of having clear and achievable treatment objectives in terms of improving people's lives. It considers the legitimate purposes of psychiatric treatment and it explores the concepts of rehabilitation and recovery. Chapter 4 draws these themes together and offers a model of strategic treatment planning.

1 Starting points

In 1981 a house physician sat on the bus on the way to work and opened the latest edition of the *British Medical Journal*. He was about to start training as a psychiatrist, so he was interested to find an editorial entitled 'The new psychiatry' (Anon., 1981). Recent research seemed to indicate that people with depressive illnesses showed neuroendocrine abnormalities that varied according to the type of depression that they were suffering from. The author was confident that in the future the use of specific and scientific tests, such as the dexamethasone suppression test, would allow more objective diagnosis of serious depression and better selection of treatment. Further research could be expected to lead to a variety of methods of measuring the physiological disturbances associated with mental illness. In the future psychiatric diagnosis would be less reliant on subjective judgements based on talking to patients. Psychiatrists, it seemed, could leave the periphery of medicine, don their white coats and enter the mainstream of the profession.

The young doctor was disheartened. He was drawn to psychiatry precisely because it involved close contact with patients and demanded a thorough understanding of their lives. The process of trying to understand patients and their problems in terms of test results and hormone assays was exactly what he disliked about general hospital medicine. His knowledge of psychiatry was absolutely rudimentary, but he was puzzled that anyone could suggest that people suffering from mental illness could be helped by a purely technological process. No matter how effectively an underlying physiological problem could be corrected, surely the human aspects of treatment would always be critical in helping the patient.

The young doctor went on to become a notoriously immodest psychiatrist. Sadly, even at this late stage, he cannot resist pointing out that he was right and that the anonymous author of the editorial was wrong. There was no breakthrough and the 'new psychiatry' never happened. Dexamethasone non-suppression is not a specific marker of severe depression. The idea that psychiatric treatment might be guided primarily by biochemical or genetic tests has not disappeared, but so far there have been no such developments of real clinical utility. Instead, clinical psychiatry has developed in a completely different, and much more constructive, direction. In our opinion, there is more cause for therapeutic optimism now than at any other time in the history of psychiatry, but that optimism does not rest on a dramatic change in the type of technical intervention available.

As the years have passed we have witnessed several similar episodes, with the announcement of an imminent or actual breakthrough in psychiatric treatment. For example, at the beginning of the 1990s rapid progress in neuroscience and the development of new drugs (the selective serotonin reuptake inhibitors and the so-called 'atypical' antipsychotics) were said to herald a new era of more effective and specific medications, which would transform the outcome of treatment. The pharmaceutical industry was so confident that a breakthrough was around the corner that it was announced that this was to be 'the decade of the CNS'. Needless to say, things did not really turn out as the industry had expected. We have yet to see a revolutionary change in clinical practice led by developments in neuroscience.

Looking back over nearly three decades of experience in mental health services, no major new treatment technologies have emerged. Certainly treatments have improved. There are many new drugs, some of which have different side effect profiles to the older medications. However, the only new medication that is demonstrably more effective than what went before is clozapine. This drug is important because it can be effective where all else fails, but there are major limitations to its usefulness. In the psychotherapies, traditional psychoanalytic approaches have been replaced by cognitive behaviour therapy and by briefer, more focused analytically based techniques. However, whilst there has been steady progress in improving psychotherapies, these techniques are essentially modifications of older technologies.

Although we recognise the limitations of technical progress we do not dismiss it. We do not point out the relative lack of technological progress in a spirit of therapeutic nihilism. On the contrary, looking back over our lengthy careers in psychiatry what is really striking is a dramatic improvement in the quality of mental health services. Whilst there is still plenty of room for improvement, interventions have become more user friendly, and the voices of patients and carers are beginning to inform both individual treatment plans and the development of services. With the slow emergence of community psychiatry we have developed new approaches to the delivery of care, such as psychiatric assertive community treatment. Most of all, the proportion of mental health professionals who are capable of forming true therapeutic alliances with patients appears to be increasing.

The old monolithic mental hospitals have closed, and as they have done so it has become increasingly apparent that, whilst the people who staffed them were largely well meaning, asylums actually caused a good deal of secondary handicap and harm. Those of us who trained in those institutions well remember the residents on the long-stay wards. They led their lives in an environment that was physically and socially bleak and impersonal. They displayed a range of deteriorated or bizarre behaviours that at the time were interpreted as symptoms of an underlying disease process, usually schizophrenia. However, as people moved out of the institutions and into smaller, homelier settings in the community, their behaviour altered. They did not suddenly stop being unwell, but many of them changed. Although some of them missed the routines and certainties of institutional life, others became more outgoing and gradually shed some of their peculiar behaviours. It seemed quite obvious to those of us who witnessed this process that some troublesome behaviours had not been symptoms of a disease at all, but a consequence of institutional care (Leff et al., 2000).

We believe that this illustrates an important general principle. Our treatment technologies, both pharmacological and psychological, are not magic bullets. They may be a necessary part of treatment, but in most situations they are not sufficient on their own to help people to overcome mental illness. The way that treatment is delivered, and the relationship between professional and patient, is absolutely critical. This is as true of the office-based treatment of a patient with depression as it is of the community treatment of someone suffering from schizophrenia. An evidence-based treatment delivered in the wrong way can cause more harm than good. Hippocrates was absolutely right to make his first injunction *do no harm*.

We believe that there are some key values and principles that underpin good clinical practice. These create the main themes in the chapters that follow. We feel that it is important to clearly state some of them here at the beginning of the book. We aim to explore the ways in which the benefits of treatment can be optimised whilst avoiding the many pitfalls that can cause harm. This is informed by our particular understanding of the legitimate role of psychiatry in patients' lives and in society at large. The nature of this legitimate role is explored in various chapters, but needless to say, it is specifically scientific in nature. This does not mean it is necessarily technological or pharmaceutical, or that it is stripped of social meaning. *'Scientific'* implies independent minded, critical and skeptical, with an awareness of the nature of evidence. Evidence can only ever be drawn from multiple sources and it is always partial and subject to revision.

In this broadly scientific spirit, what follows is based on the literature and on careful critical reflection about our own practice. We have endeavoured to understand what we do well, but also what we do poorly, and how our many mistakes have occurred. We do not suppose that we can offer a detailed programme for the reader to follow that will automatically lead to good practice. We have attempted to understand principles, but simple understanding is not enough. We have also tried to relate these principles to real and identifiable everyday practice, with all its ragged ambiguities. We have tried to avoid abstract rhetoric and thus there are many fictional clinical vignettes in what follows. In places we do identify specific treatment strategies that seem to work in some difficult clinical situations. We are well aware that before long they will become out of date, and we warn readers against slavishly following them, especially as the book ages. However, without them the book would be less useful in the real world, and what we want to do above all is to offer younger colleagues a way of developing their everyday practice without the painful process of trial and error that our own patients have had to endure.

In psychiatry, we normally think of clinical skills as interpersonal abilities that are deployed during interactions with patients. These interpersonal clinical skills are certainly extremely important. However, there are also significant intellectual clinical skills (which involve developing particular ways of thinking about problems and treatment plans) and managerial clinical skills (that are concerned with the way in which we organise our work and treatments) that are equally important. The chapters that follow explore skills in each of these three domains.

We make no apology for the reiteration of many of the themes from our previous book (Poole & Higgo, 2006), as they are critical to good practice. There are two objectives we described in that book that are especially important, because the outcome of treatment is rarely satisfactory without them:

- *Understanding context.* Mental illness occurs in a meaningful context, a personal constellation of life history, social environment and subjective experience. It is a psychiatric truism that these factors play a dominant role in causing mental illness and shaping its development. However, even when the illness is primarily biological in nature, for example, when a person has Alzheimer's disease, it is the understanding of context that allows the clinician to plan interventions that are likely to be helpful in the patient's life. Contextual understanding demands skilled history taking and observation, underpinned by an ability to empathise. This is not solely a matter of being able to appreciate what it might be like to lead a life different to one's own. Understanding context can be most difficult where the patient is similar to yourself, because there is an inevitable tendency to identify with the patient and hence overlook the important ways in which you differ.

- *Getting alongside the patient.* Psychiatric treatment works best where the professional has a relationship with the patient that is facilitative, where we support the person's ability to manage their mental disorder and hence to manage their life. Psychiatric treatment can work badly in quite a number of different ways, some of which are explored in this book. A relationship that is dominated by issues of dependency or control is bound to be of limited helpfulness, and can be positively harmful. However, dependency and control issues are bound to be present in some therapeutic relationships, either temporarily or permanently. Psychiatrists have to take responsibility for managing some aspects of risk and are often involved in treating people under compulsion. Although these roles are entirely appropriate, they can cause problems in therapeutic relationships. Even where such issues do not intrude, no therapeutic relationship can be facilitative from the outset. Getting alongside patients is a process which the psychiatrist has to manage. Therapeutic relationships that work well move from 'compliance' to 'concordance' and at any one time most relationships are in transit. Managing the journey is sometimes difficult, but it is a key clinical skill.

There are five other important ideas from our last book that we want to explain here, as readers may find our use of some words a little idiosyncratic:

- *Process.* Getting alongside the patient is just one of a number of processes that the clinician has to manage within a therapeutic relationship. All relationships have a beginning, middle and an end, and all relationships, no matter how good, can go wrong. It is not too difficult to have a good understanding of the treatment objectives within a therapeutic relationship. What takes skill is managing the process of getting there, and overcoming setbacks along the way.

- *Clinical skepticism.* Any account of one's self or someone else is affected by a range of value judgements and perceptions that can be drawn together under the heading of subjectivity. Some accounts are also influenced by a desire to withhold information or occasionally to actively mislead. Good clinicians have to maintain an attitude of skepticism, a critical and independent-minded quality that leads them to press for clarity where something does not quite make sense or where an account seems implausible ('I was cooking dinner when the argument started, and I just lashed out without noticing that the knife was in my hand'). This is not the same as being an accusatory doubting inquisitor, and it sometimes means tolerating uncertainty about the truth until it can be clarified.

- *Hypothesising.* This term is borrowed from systemic family therapy, but it is an important general clinical concept. When a psychiatrist meets a patient for the first time, before the interview starts, he invariably has a general impression of the nature of the patient's problem. This is in effect an initial clinical hypothesis. In the course of assessment, a great deal of information is gathered which leads to a more complex understanding of the individual and their problems, and the factors that have caused, shaped and sustained their difficulties. If the psychiatrist fails to clearly identify his underlying hypothesis, it is difficult to test it and to identify the features that tend to support or contradict it. Consequently, we believe that it is important to recognise clinical hypotheses, and to keep in conscious awareness the degree to which the hypothesis is supported or undermined by the facts. This includes an awareness of possible alternative hypotheses. The hypothesising process is an important part of the dialogue within mental health teams, and at an individual level should be part of discussions during supervision (we are firmly of the view that all mental health professionals should have clinical supervision, no matter how experienced or elderly they might be). Hypothesising continues throughout a therapeutic relationship, because new and important information can emerge at any time, and in any case, people's lives go on and things change. Recognising the importance of hypothesising does not imply that clinicians should dither, fail to make diagnoses or be paralysed by uncertainty. Hypothesising is the best protection against becoming so convinced of a particular way of understanding the patient that you become rigid and lead yourself into errors, either individually or, within a team, collectively. This can happen to anyone and must be actively guarded against.

- *Trajectory.* No life situation is static. Life histories and clinical problems develop and unfold under the influence of a multitude of psychological and social processes. By tracking the evolution of a situation, it is often possible to make a reasonable assessment of the likely pattern of future events. This does not amount to a detailed prediction of the future, which is always impossible. However, important tasks such as risk management can be strongly informed by, for example, the recognition of progressive social isolation, accumulating loss and the gradual extinction of hope, even where the patient truthfully denies current suicidal intentions. Furthermore, identification of an ominous trajectory can suggest interventions that might alter the person's state of well being in the long term.

- *Self-awareness.* This is difficult to achieve, and tends to fluctuate over time. Nonetheless, in order to help people with mental health problems, it is important to be aware of the impact of your own attitudes and behaviours on other people. This is important when dealing with patients, but it is also important in the interactions within teams. Gaining self-awareness rests in part on seeking accurate feedback, especially from colleagues, and receiving it without excessive defensiveness. It also requires an acknowledgement of strong personal feelings in clinical situations. Strong positive or negative feelings towards individual patients, fear or nagging apprehension over a situation or a reluctance to challenge people can all impair your clinical judgement. You have to be aware of your particular social skills and personality strengths if you are going to use them as clinical tools. Breaches of the boundaries of a professional or therapeutic relationship are most likely to be avoided if you have a good awareness of your personal vulnerabilities. You do not need years of psychotherapy in order to develop sufficient self-awareness to become, and remain, a helpful clinician, but you do need a certain openness and to pay attention to it as a long-term issue. This is another good reason for seeking clinical supervision throughout your career.

Main points in this chapter

1. In helping people suffering from mental illness, the way that psychiatric treatment is delivered is as important as the effectiveness of specific technologies.
2. Patients benefit most from professionals who can respect their autonomy and get alongside them. This does not happen automatically and the process of getting alongside patients is a skill that has to be learned.
3. We do not offer a menu of technical treatments. We explore the principles behind effective therapeutic relationships that are unlikely to change as technical treatments improve.
4. Psychiatric treatment can cause harm, even when it is delivered by competent, well-intentioned professionals.

2   A triangle of forces

Psychiatrists have a tendency to become quite excited when they are confronted with a 'classical' or 'textbook' presentation of a mental disorder. Generally speaking, clinical situations that conform closely to those described in scientific papers or great monographs seem to be the most uncommon of all presentations of mental health problems. The vast majority of people have problems that are coloured and complicated by real life, with all its multiple facets and blurred edges. In the face of this reality, one of the central challenges of mental health practice is to find rational and effective ways of intervening in situations where there is no unambiguous 'right' way of doing things.

The triangle of forces

Psychiatrists should aspire to be applied scientists, because their claim to a special credibility and expertise in helping people with mental disorders rests entirely on their scientific training. Of course, psychiatrists need to be much more than this. They especially need those essential skills that call upon their ability to empathise with other people and to understand lifestyles and mental states that are utterly different to their own. However, without access to a rational basis for intervention, we are no more useful than any other well-intentioned and empathetic member of the general public.

The trouble with this is that clinicians are constantly confronted with real situations that fall outside of the ambit of the scientific evidence, and with situations that are so complex that there is no well-established treatment pathway. The clinician has to find a way of helping people that is creative and relevant, without becoming an idiosyncratic maverick. Fortunately, the essence of being a scientist is not a comprehensive grasp of facts. Science is a way of thinking about things. There is a saying, attributed to Albert Einstein: 'Education is that which remains when one has forgotten everything one learned in school.' The most important quality of good scientists, including psychiatrists, is intellectual rigour. It is true that the profession has sometimes failed to apply sufficient skepticism to its own ideas, but this only serves to underline the importance of systematic critical reasoning as a guiding principle.

All kinds of pressures have an impact on psychiatrists' professional behaviour. However, in clinical situations there are three principle factors that can legitimately influence the decision making process. These are:
1. The scientific evidence.
2. The practitioner's clinical experience.

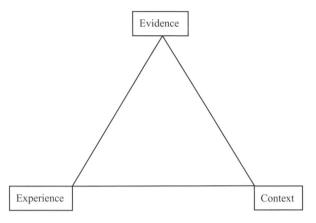

Figure 2.1 The triangle of forces.

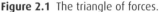

3. The practical situation, including the patient's wishes, other people's concerns, the patient's lifestyle and culture, the social environment, and realistic obstructions to the delivery of technically ideal interventions.

These can be thought of as a triangle of forces (see Figure 2.1). There are some problems with each of these factors as a primary guide to treatment. Consequently, they should remain metaphorically in a state of balance in the clinician's mind, so that he is able to establish treatment plans that are evidence based (but not mechanistic), patient centred and contextualised (but not irrational), and informed by experience (rather than by a faith in idiosyncratic ideas). Treatment frequently goes wrong because one or more of these factors has been neglected.

Scientific evidence

The powerful thing about scientific evidence is that it is systematic and reproducible. It does have intrinsic limitations. You have to understand the nature of scientific evidence in order to apply it to the task of helping people to improve their lives.

Scientific evidence is always provisional and liable to revision. It is inconceivable that mankind could ever reach the point where we knew everything about everything. Newton's laws are an accurate description of the way that the world works at the level of unassisted human observation, but they are crude and over-simplified compared to quantum physics. No matter how robust our ideas may seem at any particular point, before long they will be modified or replaced. Doctors often fall into the trap of seeming to believe that our present understanding of a disorder and its treatment is final and comprehensive. In doing this, they betray science and hence truthfulness. Part of the truth is the fact that we do not know everything, and that there are ambiguities in some aspects of every clinical situation we encounter. This is not to say that we recommend that psychiatrists embrace a post-modernist view that objective truth does not exist and that everything is relative. There is an objective truth, but it is frequently complex and hard to understand.

The truth about the effectiveness, and adverse effects, of psychiatric treatments is certainly complex. In clinical science, complexity is frequently dealt with by the use of reductionism (complexity is broken down to smaller, less complex problems) and tightly controlled methodologies (which attempt to deal with complexity by either measuring confounding variables, or eliminating complicating factors). The exemplar of this approach, whereby large numbers of people with uniform problems are treated with standardised treatments and compared in tightly controlled clinical experiments, is the randomised controlled trial (RCT). It is sometimes said that RCTs are the gold standard of evidence, but this is an oversimplification. The RCT methodology is worth thinking about because it is the dominant technology for appraising treatments at the present time, and an appreciation of some of the problems with RCTs illuminates some general issues about evidence.

RCTs are without doubt the best available methodology for isolating and assessing the effects of a specific simple treatment, such as a drug. They generate answers that are relatively statistically reliable. They have some intrinsic weaknesses. The following list is by no means comprehensive:

Firstly, RCTs generate answers that are probabilistic. We accept that a result is statistically significant if there is a one in twenty or less probability of it occurring by chance (i.e. $p \leq 0.05$). This is a convention that means that, if twenty variables are measured, at least one of them is likely to generate a statistically significant result by chance. At best, RCTs can only tell you what is likely to be true. This is the case for nearly all evidence in psychiatry, but the particular problem for RCTs is that they tend to measure large numbers of variables, and hence some results are bound to be spurious.

Secondly, in their efforts to control for complexity, RCTs are usually conducted in conditions that do not closely resemble clinical practice, on patients who have been selected for uniformity and who thus do not closely correspond to the practising psychiatrist's patient population. This creates a problem of applicability.

Thirdly, their emphasis on statistical significance can obscure the question of clinical significance. A treatment may appear to be very likely to have a particular effect, but this does not mean that the effect is of any particular importance or benefit in real life. This is the problem of relevance.

Fourthly, RCTs are difficult and expensive to conduct. They rely on statistical power, which means large numbers of subjects, which in turn leads to the involvement of multiple sites and many researchers. This introduces major problems in getting everyone to do exactly what they are meant to do in the same way. Because this is essentially impossible to achieve perfectly, data is often contaminated by hidden variability in adherence to research protocols. This may account for some of the variation in the results of different RCTs concerning the same treatment.

Fifthly, research occurs in a wider socio-economic context, which creates problems of conflict of interest. At the time of this writing there is considerable concern over the impact of pharmaceutical company sponsorship of drug trials. The majority of RCTs concerning drug treatments are sponsored by the manufacturer, and they are designed to meet the demands of regulatory authorities. There is an obvious commercial interest in positive results, and there has been growing alarm over evidence that sponsored RCTs rarely report results that are unfavourable from the company's point of view (Tungaraza & Poole, 2007). For example, the overall published evidence on antipsychotic drugs seems to show that everything is better than everything else. It appears self-evident that there is something wrong here. However, if differences between drugs are actually marginal, such findings are almost inevitable, given the intrinsic characteristics of RCTs. Whilst deliberate suppression of negative findings may happen, there are other, less sinister mechanisms by which the evidence base could be skewed. Furthermore, conflict of interest is equally important in non-RCT studies, and there are important conflicts of interest other than the commercial. Anyone who has been involved in research knows that there are major benefits for academics in finding what they want to find (not least the psychological effects of being shown to be right). Conflict of interest is a factor that needs to be borne in mind when evaluating research, but it does not necessarily invalidate findings. Gregor Mendel may have succumbed to temptation and 'improved' his results, but he retains his status as the father of genetics.

Qualitative studies have strengths and weaknesses that are the diametric opposite to those of RCTs. They have become more popular in recent years, mainly because they can explore exactly those aspects of treatment that are sacrificed in statistically robust methodologies. Asking groups of patients about their experience of treatment embraces complexity and allows an exploration of issues that are rendered invisible by the use of standardised instruments. They ask different questions to RCTs, and provide a different sort of knowledge. There is a range of other types of methodology, each with strengths and weakness, each providing evidence of a different type to a different level of reliability.

The problem with the reification of the RCT has been that it has sometimes created a sort of methodological tyranny whereby it is said that the RCT is the only type of evidence worth considering. This is misleading and unhelpful. The true gold standard of evidence is achieved when information is obtained using a range of different methodologies so that various studies, taken together, create a stereoscopic and three-dimensional picture. Of course, this does not exist as soon as a treatment becomes available; it builds over time. Evidence is an evolving process, not a question of definitive proof.

In the light of all this, there are two matching pitfalls for the practitioner. One is a slavish devotion to a vulgarised interpretation of the contemporaneous evidence. Some practitioners show a faddish predilection for the latest 'drug of choice' (or its equivalent in other therapeutic modalities). This tends to lead the practitioner to offer individual patients treatment plans that lack long-term coherence, and sometimes exposes patients to unnecessary risk. The other pitfall is scientific nihilism, a refusal to acknowledge any evidence other than that which confirms one's own prejudices. This is the royal road to charlatanism.

Clinical experience

Clinical experience is a powerful factor that shapes clinical skills, but like all other powerful things, it can be dangerous. Nearly all advances in psychiatry have originated from astute observation based on clinical experience. Aging psychiatrists who are increasingly aware of fading intellectual vigour take consolation in the belief that a depth of clinical experience has consolidated into a higher level of expertise. This may sound suspiciously like a self-serving rationalisation, but it is certainly evident as a major strength in some of our colleagues. What must be set against this is the fact that 'clinical experience' is often cited as an unverifiable justification for all sorts of questionable clinical practices. Convulsive treatments were introduced into psychiatry on the basis of the observation that epilepsy and schizophrenia rarely co-existed and therefore could be regarded as biologically antagonistic. This observation was not just wrong, it was the converse of the truth (there is an association between the two conditions) and it was only serendipity that led us to electroconvulsive treatment (ECT) as an effective treatment for severe depression and catatonia. It had nothing to do with astute clinical observation.

Given the known psychological mechanisms driving human behaviour, clinical experience is bound to exert an increasing influence on our clinical practice as the years pass. In order to use clinical experience as a creative, useful tool, it is helpful to bear some principles in mind:

- By definition, all practising clinicians are exposed to experience, but to use it you have to notice patterns, and organise what you observe. The impact of clinical experience is usually felt through an initial subjective impression. Such impressions may be a reflection of skilled observation, but they can be driven by a variety of other factors, including the clinician's own emotional reactions. One is less likely to be misled if one tries to identify the evidence for the impression. It is particularly important to remain attentive to evidence that tends to contradict such 'gut feelings'. This amounts to an application of the basic scientific method to day-to-day experience. It is easy to form impressions that are wrong, and we are ethically obliged to protect our patients from this.

- There is a constant risk of arbitrary generalisation. Sometimes this occurs because an impression is formed too quickly. An excellent example of this arises where, confronted with a new medication, the psychiatrist submits to a pharmaceutical representative's entreaties to 'try it on a few patients and see what you think'. If it is prescribed for three patients and two fail to improve, it is easy to conclude that the drug 'doesn't work'. However, such a pattern in a very small number of patients is highly likely to arise by chance. Apparently good responses or a lack of side effects are equally likely to be random phenomena. Any conclusions that are applied by the clinician to the treatment of his patients need to be based on a large enough number of observations to allow a reasonable certainty that one has noticed something real. This pitfall is a good reason for being circumspect about changes to clinical practice, especially in response to the claims of pharmaceutical representatives.

- Distressing experiences are especially potent in driving arbitrary generalisation. In the aftermath of a clinical disaster, for example, a suicide, it is entirely appropriate to carefully review the case, looking self-critically for errors, or other lessons for the future. However, to do this successfully you need to involve a third party in order to introduce a degree of objectivity. Without this, the emotional impact of the event can drive you to conclude that particular types of patients are at much higher risk than is really the case, or that some aspect of treatment has made a greater contribution to the outcome than is realistically likely. If uncontrolled, such overreactions can have adverse consequences for large numbers of patients. For example, a psychiatrist sees a sixty-four-year-old man with cognitive impairment and diagnoses Alzheimer's disease. His family finds him a residential home and sells his house, but over the next twelve months, he gradually improves. It becomes apparent that he has actually been suffering from a depressive pseudo-dementia. The patient and his family are pleased that he has recovered, but they complain because of the unnecessary changes that have been made to his circumstances on the basis of an inaccurate diagnosis. Thereafter the psychiatrist orders a brain biopsy on all patients presenting with persistent cognitive impairment. This does little to improve diagnosis, exposes subsequent patients to a degree of risk and only really serves to bolster the psychiatrist's damaged self-confidence.

- Observations that contradict one's preconceptions or psychiatric orthodoxy are more important than those that support them (except for those psychiatrists who have a temperamental tendency to be skeptical of orthodoxy, in which case the converse applies). It is always hard to admit to yourself that you are wrong, and you will not notice the evidence unless you actively look out for it.

The ability to apply lessons from clinical experience compensates for the limitations of formal scientific evidence. It is the factor that creates good or outstanding clinicians. Provided that intellectual rigour is applied to clinical experience, it is every bit as important as a grasp of the literature, if not more so. Clinical experience can teach you things that cannot be tested in formal trials. For example, best practice in rapid tranquillisation of severely disturbed patients has evolved through the application of basic pharmacology to the lessons of clinical experience. It would be difficult to conduct an ethical double-blind, placebo-controlled trial to test the effectiveness of current practice or to find staff prepared to participate in a comparison of medication with physical restraint. Furthermore, clinical experience can tell you things that then take years of research to convincingly demonstrate at a scientific level. Wing and Brown's 'three hospitals' study, published in 1970, confirmed that optimally effective rehabilitation wards were stimulating but not overly so. Many clinicians had known this for years. Indeed, there was an awareness of this in the nineteenth century and asylum superintendents tried to design rehabilitation environments accordingly (Scull, 1991). It was important to properly confirm this belief, but the finding came many years after the clinical observation.

Context

In psychiatry, context is everything. Psychopathology can only be understood with reference to the context (social as well as psychological) in which it arises. Accurate empathy is impossible without a good grasp of the patient's life circumstances. Psychiatry should be an applied science. This demands a good understanding of both the science and the situation to which it is to be applied. Standardised treatments can work, but there are all kinds of contextual factors, most importantly the patient's wishes, that mean that one has to compromise and adapt standard approaches to particular circumstances. It is essential that psychiatrists should have due regard for the patient's need for autonomy and self-respect. In doing so, one has to avoid becoming the slave of circumstantial factors.

At one level, one has to balance the demands arising from the overall situation with ethical duties and knowledge based on science and experience. Hence, prescribing an agoraphobic patient diazepam may well please him (because he will immediately feel less anxious) and his family members (because they will be able to get out and about more easily), but both experience and the evidence show that the strategy is likely to prove seriously counter-productive in the medium term. There is a serious risk that before long the patient will return to high levels of anxiety and will be burdened with the additional problems of being dependent on the drug. It is not the case that such problems are inevitable. When benzodiazepines were first introduced they were embraced as a much safer alternative to older drugs such as barbiturates. No one recognised their dependency forming properties, and behavioural approaches to anxiety problems were not widely available. Some patients with agoraphobia did remarkably well with diazepam, but most did not. Balancing the weight of the evidence with contextual factors means that, under most circumstances, diazepam is to be avoided in the treatment of agoraphobia. However, when other treatment approaches have failed and there is no realistic prospect of a successful definitive treatment, an absolute refusal to prescribe benzodiazepines can be inhumane. The problem with attending to context is that it makes it difficult to adhere to inflexible treatment algorithms (as opposed to first principles of treatment).

At another level, the difficulty with attending to context is that it can blind you to circumstances where first principles are more important than any contextual factor. The need to get alongside patients, to maintain a good quality therapeutic relationship with them, is sometimes used as reason to avoid some difficult aspect of treatment. Clinicians can become so immersed in relationship and contextual factors that they lose objectivity, and come to dismiss important risk indicators or avoid tricky tasks (for example, the raising of child protection concerns) altogether. This can only lead to incompetent and unsafe practice. In any case, a therapeutic relationship where the professional avoids an essential aspect of treatment is essentially inauthentic, and therefore seriously flawed.

No one should pretend that it is easy to understand context and get alongside patients whilst attending to difficult professional responsibilities within the relationship. However, it is not impossible, and nearly all patients appreciate and value professionals who are able to be helpful but straight talking.

Balancing the forces

Bearing these caveats in mind, the main intellectual challenge of working in mental health lies in the task of properly understanding complex situations and in creatively applying evidence and experience. This often means adapting conventional strategies, which in turn requires a sensitive understanding of how far one can go in this process before the treatment is likely to be ineffective, or irreducible first principles are likely to be broken.

The 'triangle of forces' is perhaps an oddly mechanical metaphor to use in a decidedly non-mechanical endeavour like psychiatry. We like it because we cannot think of an exception to the rule that all three factors should influence clinical practice. Most mistakes that commonly occur, from becoming overinvolved with a patient to the adoption of a sterile bio-technological approach to emotional problems, can be understood in terms of a failure of these three forces to be in balance. To over-extend the metaphorical power of Figure 2.1, you should be somewhere within the triangle at all times, well away from the edges and certainly nowhere near the corners. The responsibility for maintaining this position lies entirely with the practitioner. Many external agencies exert pressure to ignore one or two of these forces. Pharmaceutical companies, policy makers, misguided relatives of patients, hospital managers, insurers and others have an interest in deflecting the clinician to one corner or another. Each of these deflecting influences has a prima facie validity, and these pressures can be hard to resist. The ability to steer an appropriate course is one of the marks of a good clinician. It is based on personal integrity, the most important component of professionalism.

Main points in this chapter

1. Psychiatrists' claim to special expertise in helping people suffering from mental disorder arises solely from their scientific training.
2. The essence of science is intellectual rigour and, as far as possible, psychiatrists need to apply this to all areas of their practice.
3. Evidence, experience and context are the principle factors that legitimately influence clinical decision making.
4. It is the professional's responsibility to hold these three 'forces' in balance.

3 Treatment objectives

What is psychiatric treatment for?

This question is not a philosophical abstraction, nor is the answer self-evident. There are ambiguities embedded in all medical practice concerning the purpose of treatment. They arise from the fact that there are major differences between suffering and symptoms, between disease and illness, and between getting better and feeling well. Few of us can get through life without discovering that the experience of medical treatment is sometimes more unpleasant than the illness itself.

Policy makers and their de facto partners, the media, seem to take the position that mental health services can only be regarded as successful if they eliminate mental illness completely from the public arena. This is incompatible with what is possible and with the values of the mental health community, which is the loose coalition of mental health professionals, voluntary groups, service users and carers who have a continuous interest in mental health. The consensus view within it is that the quality of life of people suffering from mental illness would improve considerably if the rest of the population were to become more tolerant of difference, and more accepting of the fact that there will always be mentally ill people living amongst them. Everyone wishes to avoid serious adverse consequences of mental illness, including suicide, violence and self-neglect. However, policy makers and the mental health community differ over the appropriateness of strict enforcement of flawed and only partially effective treatment technologies.

Government policies cannot be completely ignored, but it appears that we cannot rely on policy makers to help us find sensible answers to questions regarding the legitimate purpose of psychiatric treatment. It has taken mental health services a very long time to get around to asking people who suffer from mental illness what they would like to achieve through accepting psychiatric treatment. This might seem like the obvious thing to do. However, until quite recently there has been a reluctance to take patients' opinions seriously, on the basis that those opinions might be irrational or lack coherence. In fact, now that mental health services have finally started to listen to service users' opinions, it is clear that the things they want are consistent and entirely reasonable, but that there are significant differences in emphasis to the priorities identified by clinicians (Perkins, 2001).

The only legitimate objective of treatment is to improve people's lives. This may involve reducing or eliminating symptoms. Sometimes it involves accepting that symptoms cannot be eliminated, but finding ways of having a better life despite them.

Box 3.1 Escape from the revolving door

Ken was a fifty-five-year-old man who suffered from a recurrent schizoaffective disorder. He first became unwell at the age of thirty-five, when he was working as a journalist on a regional newspaper. Ken was a man with strong political opinions, who had been heavily involved in the anti-nuclear movement. When ill, he believed that he was under surveillance by the CIA, and felt that he had a responsibility to take direct action to stop injustices in the world. In the past he had attempted to gain access to 10 Downing St, Buckingham Palace and the American Embassy. He responded well to treatment, but he was consistent in his refusal to accept it other than under legal compulsion. When well he would acknowledge that his actions had been ill advised, but he attributed this to understandable outrage rather than mental illness. He insisted that he only wanted to talk to powerful people. He denied any intention to harm them.

Ken's refusal to accept treatment meant that there were recurrent episodes of disinhibited and alarming behaviour. His marriage broke down and he lost his job. He spent all his savings and he lived in a small bedsit in a run down area. He was admitted to hospital every year. When well, he teasingly accused the mental health services of being agents of a corrupt state. When ill, he angrily believed they were acting under the direction of the US State Department. On admission to hospital he was given depot antipsychotic medication. He accepted this for a few months after discharge, but would complain that he could not concentrate. When he refused the medication, his concentration would improve. There would be a period during which he would get some writing done. This would be followed by relapse and readmission. His quality of life was poor, a cycle of illness and remission which revolved too quickly to ever allow him to regain anything that he had lost as a consequence of his illness.

Things changed in Ken's life as a result of concerns about national security in the aftermath of 11th September 2001. Previously his attempts to get in touch with prominent people had been perceived as a nuisance. In the new atmosphere of heightened tension, his next attempt to gain access to the American Embassy resulted in him being apprehended at gunpoint, followed by interrogation by anti-terrorist police officers. When the police released him to the care of the mental health service, they warned that he had been lucky. If he behaved like this again, there was a significant risk that he would be shot.

The existing pattern of treatment was no longer appropriate. Unless something changed, Ken would be at risk of serious harm. He was referred to the assertive outreach team. They were able to sustain a high level of contact with Ken. They recognised that he would not accept continuous medication, and so they struck an agreement with him. They would not press medication, provided he accepted visits three times a week. They would concentrate on reducing the stresses in his life, and on identifying warning signs that he was entering an acute episode. If they saw signs of this they would offer him medication, and if he refused this they would apply a low threshold for compulsory readmission.

Initially the plan failed, and Ken was quickly back in hospital, albeit without a faux pas outside of a high profile address. After this, however, things changed. Ken accepted visits. When he started to become unwell, he accepted oral medication, though only for a few weeks. He was helped to find better accommodation, and he was encouraged to work on his writing. Unimpaired by either hospital admissions or drug side effects, he managed to get a regular column in a local newspaper. He did not accept that he suffered from a mental illness, and most of the time he was chronically over-expansive. However, he came to acknowledge that the mental health services were on his side and that life had improved.

The previous treatment objective had been implicit and unstated. It had been to get Ken to accept medication in order to stop him from getting ill. There was no realistic possibility that he would agree to this. The new treatment objective was to avoid circumstances where his behaviour would get him shot and to help him to achieve the things that he wanted for himself. The first treatment plan had failed. The second succeeded through a combination of co-operation, duress and toleration of low-grade symptoms.

If psychiatric treatment does not give people a better life than they would have without treatment, then it is both ineffective and unethical. Improving people's lives is a challenging objective. It is hard enough to assess how particular symptoms are likely to respond to specific interventions. It is harder still to reliably predict how this will affect the person's daily life. Clinicians tend to focus their attention on problems in peoples' brains or minds. This is a consequence of our training and professional cultures, and there is nothing wrong with it provided that it helps to resolve problems in patients' lives. If therapies aimed at altering minds or brains have no positive impact on people's lives, then they are essentially worthless. The most important questions we ask people are not 'how have you been feeling?' or 'how are the voices?' but 'what have you been doing with your time?' and 'what do you plan to do?' The balance of beneficial and adverse effects of intervention must be assessed in the arena of everyday activity, because for most people it is their life as it is lived that really matters to them.

We believe that the link between treatment objectives and improvement in peoples' lives is a necessary condition for successful treatment. It has no exceptions. However, one cannot deny that there are problems and paradoxes. For example, who is to make the God-like judgement that a particular treatment is likely to have a positive effect on the person's life? Clearly the patient's opinion on the matter has the greatest claim to validity, but he may not be in a good position to judge. Furthermore, psychiatrists and other mental health professionals spend a good part of their working lives trying to get people to do things they do not want to do. People who want to be in hospital are persuaded to stay at home, while people who want to stay at home are persuaded to accept admission. People are urged to confront those things that frighten them the most and which they most want to avoid. People who do not want medication are persuaded to take drugs, whilst people who like taking drugs are encouraged to stop. There seems to be an underlying principle of treatment that, according to mental health services, whatever you want is the opposite of what is good for you. Sometimes we believe this so strongly that we force people to do things they do not want to do. Somehow, for this to be justified, it still has to lead to an eventual improvement in the person's life.

The normal ethical justification for the use of compulsion is that patients are unable to understand their situation properly as a consequence of their illness (in other words they lack mental capacity with regard to treatment). It is assumed that if they did understand, they would agree with the professionals' decisions. In due course most people get better, and in real life some people who have experienced compulsory treatment come to agree that it was the right thing under the circumstances. Some patients, however, do not. Even after they get better, they continue to object and to hold a different opinion to the professionals. Some patients do not recover at all. They remain unwell and incarcerated indefinitely in psychiatric facilities. These patients are relatively few in number, but their treatment poses an important ethical dilemma. It is hard to argue that treatment is improving their lives, but failure to treat seems seriously neglectful. If the patient *never* comes to agree that treatment has improved his life, can the treatment be regarded as appropriate or ethical?

Long-term compulsory treatment is most usually justified on the grounds that an improvement in the patient's life is likely to come about eventually and that a collaborative approach is impossible. One can also justify compulsory treatment in order to avoid adverse consequences for the patient, in other words, to prevent a deterioration in the person's life. This usually concerns risk management, including the risk that the person will act violently and suffer consequences at the hands of the criminal justice system. However, these are progressively more uncertain treatment objectives, which rest upon the unreliable and inexact science of predicting people's behaviour. We need to guard against unwittingly straying into a situation where we are making the patient's life worse, not better. In order to avoid repetition of psychiatry's historical errors in this regard, we have to try to be clear about treatment objectives.

Rehabilitation and recovery

The concept of rehabilitation is presently unfashionable, but it remains an important method of organising the task of improving people's lives. The word has some difficult resonances, as 'rehabilitation' has sometimes been used as a euphemism for warehousing people with severe mental illness in barren and deteriorated environments, and engaging them in repetitive and inane activity. 'Habilitation' would be a more accurate term. According to the Shorter Oxford English Dictionary (SOED) this means 'the action of enabling'. This better captures the aim of the process, and embraces not only the restoration of abilities that have been lost, but also the gaining of skills and a quality of life that the person has never previously experienced. However, 'rehabilitation' is the internationally recognised term, and so we shall use it.

Rehabilitation is a stepwise process, whereby each stage in treatment is not an end in itself, but a step towards a long-term aim. Not everyone suffering from mental illness needs rehabilitation, but the concept is applicable to the treatment of a significant proportion of people with mental health problems. Its importance is certainly not confined to the treatment of those suffering from chronic psychosis. Rehabilitationists have come to recognise that special, sheltered facilities for the mentally ill have a limited role in the process. The problem with them is that they easily become a dead end, acculturating the person to a life of permanent separation from the rest of the community. Rehabilitation is most meaningful when it happens amongst society in general, where the person can be part of the ordinary things in life. If rehabilitation has to start in separate or parallel facilities, this can only be a prelude to the process. In the UK the term 'social inclusion' has been misused by politicians to the point where it has taken on a euphemistic quality, but stripped of these overtones, it exactly captures what rehabilitation is all about. It is a high-level treatment objective.

It is extraordinary that the word 'recovery' has only recently entered the general vocabulary of mental health services. One might have supposed that recovery was always the implicit objective of psychiatric treatment. In fact there is no doubt that for many service users one of the most difficult aspects of being part of the mental health system was the implicit assumption that recovery was not a possibility and that they had to accept a lifetime of dependency on professionals. Although none of us intended to be so pessimistic, it is hardly surprising that our patients came to feel that we were extinguishing hope of a normal life. It was the service user movement that first asserted that recovery was an important and achievable treatment objective. The increasing acceptance of this within the mental health community has had a major impact on the development of services. We should not have been so slow to listen properly to what our patients were telling us (Roberts & Wolfson, 2004).

The essence of recovery is that the person gains, or is restored to, a state of personal autonomy and a sense of well being. It does not mean a denial of the recurrent or chronic nature of some mental illnesses. One of the big problems with being mentally ill is that you can find yourself with little control over your life. Your life can come to be controlled by the illness, or by professionals, or both. Mental illness can leave people with a permanent sense of being impaired and vulnerable, whether symptoms are present or not. Recovery is a realistic expectation even for people with severe and chronic illness. Where people cannot recover fully, they can recover partially. Recovery can mean discharge from services and discontinuation of treatment, but these are not prerequisite. With or without professional support it means having a degree of mastery over the illness and its treatment. It requires that professionals get alongside patients and help them to learn to manage their own illness. There is no conceivable rating scale or clinical instrument that can measure recovery. People have recovered when they feel that they have got their life back.

Although the recognition by mental health services that recovery is an important treatment objective is a relatively new development, there are already signs that the concept is open to abuse. Some services claim to be working to 'the Recovery Model'. There is no such model. Recovery is an objective, and there are many different routes to achieve it. The Recovery Model can be a thin rationalisation for the withdrawal of services. The logic goes something like this: if dependency on services is a bad thing because it impedes recovery, then the person will be better off and more likely to recover if services are withdrawn. The inevitable result is that some people are left without the support they need and their lives get worse. The organisation, however, has found a righteous way of saving money.

Where recovery is held as a treatment objective in every case, there is bound to be a significant alteration in the way that mental health services function and in service users' experience of treatment. Many people have been in mental health services for decades, and they can find such a dramatic change of attitude difficult. A degree of dependency is an almost inevitable consequence of an intervention that the person finds helpful. Dependency can be resolved, but it can take some time. Unrealistic expectations are not the route to recovery. Therapeutic optimism that is robust in the face of setbacks, on the other hand, is essential. The clinician has to work with patients to understand what would have to happen for them to feel that they had recovered, and how to get there. Needless to say, working towards recovery requires a shared appreciation of risks and risk taking.

Getting alongside patients does not necessarily mean doing everything they want. To return to the example from Chapter 2, some people want to be given benzodiazepines when they feel anxious. For the majority of people there are better, though slower solutions, including tolerating anxiety. Anxiety passes and it is an inevitable part of life. Simply doing what patients want is likely to be counter-productive, because they would not need to see a psychiatrist if they knew what to do, or if the methods they have been using to cope hitherto had worked. To achieve recovery, patients need professionals who are upfront and honest, who can openly discuss difficult matters, who can respect them and their point of view, and who can share their expertise in such a way that it is transferred and becomes part of the patient's repertoire for dealing with their problems.

Who benefits from psychiatric treatment?

Experienced mental health professionals tend to have a good empathic understanding of other people. They can readily understand how emotional problems arise, and they can make sense of experiences that appear senseless and distressing to the person who is suffering from them. They can understand antecedents and they can reframe problems in a helpful way. As there is no clear boundary between mental illness and ordinary emotional distress, they can put their skills to use in helping people who are suffering from a wide range of emotional difficulties and mental disorders. However, just because they can make interventions with people suffering from problems of all levels of intensity (from being upset through to being severely psychotic) does not mean that they should go ahead and do so.

There is an old joke about Woody Allen: 'Thirty-five years in psychoanalysis and then he marries his step-daughter; you'd ask for your money back!' We have never met Mr Allen, his wife or his psychoanalyst, and in all probability the implications in the joke are entirely unfair. However, there is an important point here. The indiscriminate use of mental health interventions is not necessarily appropriate or useful.

We were working in Liverpool in 1989 when the Hillsborough disaster happened. Liverpool Football Club was playing a cup match in Sheffield. In order to avoid violence in the crowd, their supporters (predominantly Liverpool residents) were corralled into a fenced enclosure, the Leppings Lane End, with no escape routes. Owing to poor crowd control, an abnormally severe pressure of people occurred on the terrace, and 96 people were crushed to death. The match was televised live, and families sat and watched helplessly at home, knowing that loved ones were involved in the unfolding tragedy.

This was not the first disaster at a football match. Following the received wisdom of the time, the city council decided to contact every survivor who had been in the Leppings Lane End and to offer them counselling, in the belief that this would prevent them from developing long-term emotional problems. There was disquiet about this response amongst mental health professionals in the city, not least because it involved a diversion of resources from other priorities. However, there was a general feeling abroad in Liverpool that this was the appropriate thing to do. There was no clear evidence for the efficacy of this approach at the time, and subsequently it has been shown that psychological debriefing can make a poor emotional adjustment more likely (Kenardy, 2000). Although teams of counsellors continue to be sent to work with traumatised populations, a significant body of opinion holds that the best practice is to allow people to experience natural and unavoidable distress, in the knowledge that most people will recover from it. People are resilient and if they have the necessary support and personality resources, the solutions they find to their problems will often be better than professionally mediated solutions. Of course, some people for one reason or another will be persistently distressed, and then there are good grounds for intervention.

Antidepressants and psychotherapy can relieve emotional distress, but there is a high cost for individuals and communities if they come to be seen as inevitable and necessary in order to overcome the distress caused by problems of life. Life is intrinsically a distressing business. It is full of loss and injustice. As a society we seem perilously close to the view that distress is a disorder and that people should not be allowed to experience it. However, distress, anxiety and anger are normal emotions that can spur constructive change. Everyone's autonomy and well being is undermined if we come to feel that the only appropriate response to difficult feelings is to have them eliminated by professionals (Summerfield, 2004).

If the primary goal of psychiatric treatment is to improve people's lives, this has to be tempered by the constraint that psychiatric treatment should only be undertaken if the person is unlikely to recover on a similar timescale without it. Even where an intervention is necessary, there are often other respectable non-psychiatric ways of securing help. Voluntary sector organisations can be better at helping people with some types of problem than psychiatrists are. In the UK, and throughout the developed world, there are voluntary organisations that have expertise in helping people with bereavement, marital problems, addictions and a range of other difficulties. They have the advantage of being more closely embedded in local communities than mental health services. They are also cheaper. Even where mental health care is a market commodity, there is not an infinite supply. Psychiatric expertise is a finite resource in any society, and it should be targeted on those who benefit most, no matter where funding comes from.

Finally, psychiatrists should not attempt to treat conditions where they have little or nothing to offer. People whose problems fall outside of the scope of psychiatry often end up under mental health services by default. For example, people of normal intelligence with autistic spectrum disorders can find themselves under generic mental health services for lack of an obvious alternative source of help. In fact, other resources do exist that are better able to deal with the essentially developmental nature of their problems, but you have to know how to access them. Once in mental health services there is a tendency to treat such people as if they have a mental illness, which often means the inappropriate use of psychotropic medication or misguided efforts to deploy psychological or social interventions that are designed to help people with entirely dissimilar difficulties.

There are well-recognised hazards in heroic attempts to treat people with intractable personality difficulties. The fact of being under psychiatric care can be used to avoid normal penalties for anti-social behaviour. In this way, fruitless treatment can unwittingly reinforce exactly the behaviours that it is supposed to eliminate. However, we should emphasise that there are real grey areas and that we are not suggesting that either diagnosis or 'treatability' should be exclusive criteria for psychiatric treatment. It can be difficult to determine whether someone is deriving benefit that could not be obtained in any other way. Whilst it is generally true that mental health services are best at helping people suffering from mental illnesses such as schizophrenia, bipolar affective disorder and major depression, there are conditions that are neither treatable in the traditional sense nor strictly speaking mental illnesses that do fall appropriately within the ambit of psychiatry. For example, many men suffering from pathological jealousy seem to suffer not so much from a mental illness but rather personality difficulties that are characterised by insecure attachment. This is usually true even where jealousy is delusional. Jealousy in all its forms is notoriously difficult, if not impossible, to eliminate. Some would say that it is fundamentally an untreatable problem. However, involvement with mental health services over a period of time can help people to contain their feelings and to reduce the well-recognised risk of serious violence. Although disengagement and a return to a dangerously volatile situation is common, such interventions can be relatively successful, and there is usually no other agency that can more appropriately carry out the task.

Mental health services have to be able to help people with a wide range of problems beyond their mental illness. For example, about thirty percent of people suffering from schizophrenia have a substance misuse problem and the figure is even higher for bipolar affective disorder (Ferrier *et al.*, 2001; McCreadie, 2002). Mental health services have to be able to work with these problems, because addiction services can find mental illness difficult to manage, and in any case, the frequency of the problem is so high that it can be regarded as part of the mental illness syndromes. Even services that are closely focussed on those patients suffering from severe mental illness have to have the capacity to deal with difficulties outside of this narrow remit if they are to improve people's lives.

Psychiatry can legitimately treat people with the whole range of mental disorders, from schizophrenia to anorexia nervosa, from depression to personality disorder, and from obsessive-compulsive disorder to drug dependence. However, patients should always be likely to derive some benefit that they could not have obtained in another way.

Main points in this chapter

1. Mental illnesses affect peoples' lives, and it is improvement in peoples' lives that marks successful treatment.
2. Recovery does not imply a denial of the recurrent or long-term nature of many mental health problems. It is characterised by regaining personal autonomy and a sense of well being.
3. Treatment objectives should be explicit and shared.
4. Psychiatric treatment should only be undertaken if the patient is unlikely to experience a timely recovery without it.
5. Psychiatric treatment should not be undertaken if there is more appropriate expertise available elsewhere.

4 Strategic treatment

Good psychiatric treatment is helpful, relevant and safe, and the balance of personal cost–benefit for the patient is positive. There are two fundamental skills needed to achieve this (Poole & Higgo, 2006). The first is the ability to carry out a good quality assessment that leads to an understanding of the factors that have led *this* patient to develop *these* symptoms at *this* time. It involves much more than making a diagnosis. Equally as important is the ability to elicit and understand the full range of contextual factors (psychological, social and biological) that are affecting the person. The second is the ability to form, over time, a particular type of therapeutic alliance with the patient, what we have called getting alongside patients.

The next critical step in achieving good treatment is what you actually do, those specific interventions that attempt to solve problems. A well-conducted assessment will give the psychiatrist a picture of the key problems affecting the patient. These tend to be interrelated, and frequently play against a backdrop of themes in people's lives, such as their characteristic patterns of coping with difficulties (largely determined by their personality) and issues determined by culture, personal beliefs, and family or occupational environment. The clinician does not just have to select the right interventions from the menu of potential treatments. Treatment has to make sense to the patient, interventions have to be sequenced and the overall package has to have a coherence that leads it towards identifiable objectives.

Treatment can proceed reactively or strategically. In our experience, the strategic approach is far more effective. We believe that the difference between the two approaches probably accounts for much of the variation in effectiveness between different clinicians of apparently similar ability. There are many pressures that may lead even the best clinicians towards a reactive approach. Reactive treatment tends to come more naturally to doctors. Doctors like to do things, and this can lead them to do far too much. At best this means that they do things that are unnecessary. Over time it can create a real incoherence in the overall pattern of treatment. In order to avoid this, it is useful to bear in mind the principles underlying strategic approaches to treatment. These are:

- Forming a shared understanding of the nature of the problem.
- Clarity over the objectives and limitations of treatment.
- Prioritising problems, sharing the overall plan and proceeding in a stepwise fashion.
- Anticipating setbacks, and evaluating them when they occur.
- Knowing when to stick to the plan and when to change it.

- Maintaining realistic therapeutic optimism.
- Recognising when enough has been achieved.

Before exploring these principles, we should perhaps clarify what strategic and reactive treatment look like in practice.

A commonplace clinical scenario

Mr Kennedy was a thirty-six-year-old man who was referred to Dr Jackson suffering from depression. He had had a settled and happy suburban childhood, and he did well at school. At university he gained a good degree in chemical engineering, and went on to a job in the chemical industry. By the age of twenty-nine he was married with two small children, and his career was progressing well. He was promoted away from a technical role into a management position, and his employers indicated that they felt that he had a bright future.

By the age of thirty-four he was the general manager of a medium-sized chemical plant, and he was struggling. He found personnel issues difficult, because he disliked conflict. The company was pressing for higher productivity, which the staff organisa-tions resisted. The twin imperatives of safety and productivity were in conflict with each other, and he became increasingly worried about the risk of an industrial accident. He started drinking in the evenings in order to relax, which angered his wife who pressed him to become more involved with the family. He was caught in a cycle of stress at work and conflict at home. Two months before his referral, his worst fears came to fruition and there was an accidental release of several tons of toxic gas from the plant. He led the major incident response. No one was harmed, but for three days the local press hounded him. His press statement was selectively quoted in the paper, and he was identified as the person responsible for jeopardising the health of local children. He went to see his general practitioner (GP), who signed him off sick and referred him to a psychiatrist, Dr Jackson.

On assessment, Dr Jackson found that Mr Kennedy was moderately depressed, with loss of appetite and weight, sleep disturbance and impaired concentration. He was angry with his employers who he felt had put him in an impossible position and then left him to carry the can when things went wrong. He knew that the press had exaggerated the health risks attributable to the accident, but felt that the local community now saw him as a monster. He feared that he would be recognised in the street, and that he might even be attacked. He could not face the thought of returning to work, and felt that his career was now destroyed. Anticipating the sack, he felt shame at the prospect of his family living in reduced circumstances. He was avoiding looking at bills and bank statements, because he feared that the family faced eventual financial ruin. He was drinking a bottle of wine each night, sometimes followed by brandy. His wife was worried, and there were frequent arguments over his morose withdrawal, his drinking, his refusal to deal with routine finances and his insistence that the family would be better off without him. He denied suicidal thoughts, but he readily stated that he saw no future for himself.

For Dr Jackson, this generated the following problem list:

1. Moderately depressed, with significant risk of developing suicidal ideas.
2. High level of alcohol intake over several years, increasing recently. Alcohol problem well established but probably secondary to stress at work. Some increase in tolerance to the effects of alcohol but no other evidence of physical dependency.
3. Intelligent man with marked degree of obsessionality, though no frank obsessional symptoms. Personality well suited to technical job, less suited to frontline management position. Self-esteem and self-confidence significantly damaged prior to accident, now very poor. Consequently, catastrophising his situation.
4. Coping with this by avoidance and withdrawal from life.
5. Acute on chronic marital problem.

A reactive approach to the situation

Faced with this list of interrelated difficulties on first assessment, Dr Jackson could reasonably (but misguidedly) immediately arrange the following interventions:

1. Mr Kennedy was moderately depressed with biological features and some hopelessness. The degree and pattern of depression was such that one could reasonably expect a good response to antidepressant treatment. An SSRI would be the best choice, as these drugs are not sedative, and the risk of dangerous interaction with alcohol would be minimised. Prescribe fluoxetine 20 mg once a day.
2. Despite the fact that the heavy drinking was not the primary problem, a referral to the local alcohol treatment unit could be justified on the grounds that problem drinking was now well established, and probably exacerbating depression, sleep disturbance and marital discord. Refer to alcohol service.
3. There were current issues regarding negative self-image, catastrophisation and avoidance, combined with longer term issues relating to coping strategies and occupational choices. These were all within the scope of cognitive behaviour therapy (CBT). Refer to CBT nurse therapist.
4. There were real problems within the marriage that had been building up for some years. Marital therapy is difficult if one partner is identified as the 'patient' and therefore has the primary relationship with the service. It is better for the couple to refer themselves for joint help from a separate specialist agency. Recommend self-referral to local voluntary sector marriage guidance organisation.

The problem with this approach is that it lacks coherence. The psychiatrist has simply identified a series of problems, and reacted to all of them. There is nothing wrong with any of the individual interventions, but they are not prioritised and sequenced. Because of this, each intervention is less likely to be effective. The effectiveness of the antidepressant is likely to be undermined by a high alcohol intake until this is under control. Marital therapy is likely to focus on Mr Kennedy's drinking and depression if these have shown no change at the point of intervention. CBT is unlikely to be effective in the presence of heavy drinking. There is a mixed message with regard to its likely effectiveness in the face of the implied 'belt and braces' of a simultaneous prescription of an antidepressant. Mr Kennedy may take the implication from multiple interventions that everything about him (his brain, his mind, his self-control and his marriage) has gone wrong and needs fixing. Furthermore, his ability to find his own solutions to some problems may be undermined by the clear message that the way forward is mainly through professional help.

Despite these drawbacks, this approach can be successful some of the time. However, there is a further weakness, in that it is difficult to find a creative way forward if things do not go well. The referrals may lead to significant delays or Mr Kennedy may be reluctant to go along with some part of the plan. Even if there is a timely response to requests for specialist intervention and Mr Kennedy accepts all the advice that he has been given, he may not show immediate signs of improvement. It certainly would be difficult for him to gives his full attention to the separate interventions of four different professionals, even if his concentration had been unimpaired in the first place. For any of these reasons, Dr Jackson might well find no sign of improvement six weeks after initial assessment. Whether he says so or not, Mr Kennedy might well feel that any glimmer of hope that he gained after his first appointment was extinguished by the disappointment of an evident lack of change. The trouble is Dr Jackson would not have a Plan B. In the face of an unchanged or deteriorating clinical situation, his alternatives would lie between doing nothing (which is difficult within a reactive approach because it implies that the clinician is indifferent or impotent), admitting the patient to hospital (which might have been unnecessary with a more systematic approach, and which Mr Kennedy may well be reluctant to accept) or changing the medication. Under these circumstances, there is a law of diminishing returns; each sequential medication change is less likely to be effective than the previous one, and there is a real danger of sliding into polypharmacy and a fruitless search for the magic medication (or more commonly the magic cocktail of medications) that will unlock the situation. The only people who are likely to benefit from this situation are psychiatrists who run specialist tertiary services, because the victims of this type of incoherent treatment are their bread and butter.

A strategic approach

There is another way. Firstly, Dr Jackson feeds back to Mr Kennedy his understanding of the situation. Although Mr Kennedy has told the story, even psychologically sophisticated people often fail to recognise what is happening to them when they become depressed. By feeding back, the problem is reframed and the main message in Mr Kennedy's case is that he has developed a depressive illness in the face of understandable stressors that might have a similar effect on many people. Furthermore, although it all looks very gloomy at the moment, there is a plausible way forward. One part of the discussion might involve Dr Jackson saying something like:

> You are depressed, and this has reached the point where low mood sustains itself. Although you may feel that alcohol is helping, it is a powerful depressant and is undoubtedly contributing to the problem. The trouble with being depressed is that it leads you to construe things in the most negative possible way. The publicity about the incident is distressing but, as they say, today's news is tomorrow's fish

and chip paper, and it is unlikely that the community will remember your part in the incident. Once you are feeling a bit better, we need to think about your job, but it's too soon to decide whether you should do anything about it or not. However, it does sound as if we'll need to think about how you cope with stress. Similarly, your marriage may improve as you feel better, but it's possible you will need some help as a couple to improve your relationship.

   The first thing to do is to stop drinking, and I want you to keep an alcohol diary, so that, if you do drink, we can understand the triggers. If you do stop, then your mood is likely to improve significantly within a week or so. If you cannot stop, antidepressant treatment is unlikely to work, but in any case your alcohol problem may be worse than I think, and we may need to get some specialist help. It's likely that we'll decide that you should take an antidepressant in due course, but we'll do things one step at a time.

This creates a treatment plan that has an understandable rationale and an overarching strategy. There are some simple and specific tasks for Mr Kennedy to perform that give him some control over his recovery. If things do not work at any stage, Dr Jackson has retained a range of further options. Importantly, he will intervene as it proves necessary, avoiding a counter-productive therapeutic overkill. Each appointment can be focussed on particular tasks that contribute to the overall objectives (for example, the next appointment will be focussed on his drinking and, if he is abstinent, the extent of any improvement). Dr Jackson has endeavoured to instil realistic hope that the situation will improve whilst acknowledging that some problems may persist and may or may not demand attention in their own right.

Such an approach does mean that it is usually necessary to see patients relatively frequently at first, but this is offset by the fact that there is a good chance that the intensity of medium-term input will be reduced.

Forming a shared understanding of the nature of the problem

There are very few good reasons to avoid being frank with patients, but explaining your understanding of patients' problems in a way that they can easily comprehend does take some skill. At one level one has to adjust vocabulary to accommodate to the patient's level of education. Some concepts that are very familiar to a mental health professional, such as depression or schizophrenia, are very poorly understood by a large proportion of the general public, and this means that these diagnoses have to be explained. Baldly stating that someone has a depressive illness conveys little information unless one explains the nature of such illnesses in some detail. Some terms, such as the expression 'clinical depression' or a DSM/ICD number generally cause confusion rather than clarity. It is usually helpful to frame explanations with reference to the effects on everyday life and relate information to the patient's own circumstances. No one finds it easy to make sense of abstract information.

   There is often a temptation to use euphemisms or to otherwise slide away from difficult issues, especially those concerning risk. Needless to say, this temptation is to be avoided. Risk has a major role in decision making, and if a risk issue is not explained to patients, they are likely to find your behaviour hard to understand. Discussing the risk of self-harm is usually fairly straight forward, because it is part of routine assessment. What is sometimes overlooked is involving patients in managing the risk of self-harm. Many (but not all) patients consider suicide because they can see no way forward, and it can be important to discuss this and to explore whether the person finds the treatment plan plausible. Your expectation of change on a tolerable (and stated) timescale can significantly affect the patient's sense of being hopeless and helpless. Telling someone that you think they are at risk of harming someone else, and how you think this should be managed, is altogether more challenging, but it is essential to do it.

It is the shared nature of the understanding of the problem that is important, and sometimes this involves more than the mental health professional simply explaining to the patient how it is. There is a range of circumstances where the patient and the psychiatrist have markedly different ideas about the nature of the problem. For example, a psychotic patient's belief that his misfortunes are due to persecution at the hands of the Russian Mafia cannot be easily reconciled with the psychiatrist's belief that the patient is suffering from schizophrenia, and similarly a person who is depressed and hypochondriacal may find it impossible to accept that the problem is fundamentally psychological rather than physical in nature.

Fortunately, a shared understanding does not rest on complete agreement about everything. It can include a recognition that the psychiatrist and the patient have markedly different ideas about the cause (or some other aspect) of the problem. Under most circumstances, doctor and patient agree about much more than they disagree about, and this usually allows a shared understanding that acknowledges and accommodates differences. This is not the same as colluding with bizarre or palpably incorrect ideas; it is more a question of respecting the other person's right to be wrong.

There will always be some circumstances where the psychiatrist and the patient can find no common understanding of the problem, for example, when someone is being treated for mania under compulsion and they simply do not believe that there is anything wrong at all. These situations are relatively uncommon, and are usually fairly transient. It is then the process of working towards a shared understanding that is important.

Under many circumstances, especially where the patient is suffering from a more serious and enduring mental illness, the relationship between the mental health team and the patient's family is important. Developing a shared understanding of the problem with a family, especially where there are complications such as persistent substance misuse, takes considerable time and effort. It can be a complex task, given families' well-known tendency to harbour tension and disagreement. However, the development of a sophisticated understanding with the family can make an enormous difference to the patient's well being.

Clarity over the objectives and limitations of treatment

We explored the issue of treatment objectives at length in Chapter 3, and only a few points need to be added here. Generally speaking, treatment objectives tend to fall out of a shared understanding of the problem. Objectives have to be formed in the awareness of the limitations of treatment. On the whole, successful psychiatric treatments facilitate changes in people's lives. Helping someone's depression to lift changes the way that they behave. Mental health problems tend to arise as a consequence of a downward spiral of accumulating problems, worsening symptoms and poor coping strategies. Treatments tend to work where they allow the process to reverse, with an upward spiral of renewed optimism, changes in behaviour and reciprocal changes in other people's attitudes and behaviours. There are very few circumstances where the patient recovers entirely as a direct effect of the treatment itself. Indeed, one of the patterns of treatment failure involves an initial improvement but no tangible alteration in the person's life circumstances. There is then a deterioration as initial hope turns to disillusionment.

It follows that patients need to be aware of the facilitative nature of psychiatric treatment from the outset. It is easy to unwittingly set up expectations that are unrealistic, and which are likely to cause significant problems when they are not fulfilled. Antidepressants cannot resolve chronic unhappiness over life circumstances, and psychotherapies cannot remake personalities or undo traumatic life experiences. It is not the case that chronically unhappy lives cannot improve, or that people with personality problems cannot be helped, or that people cannot come to feel differently about awful events. However, the work of overcoming these things belongs primarily to the person suffering from them, and some of this work cannot be planned programmatically by the professional. Our role is usually to help people to modify small but important bits of behaviour, to help them to do things slightly differently, in the knowledge that the effects of such changes tend to amplify over time. In our experience there is an important principle here: in general, people start to feel differently when they do things differently. It does sometimes happen that emotional change precedes behavioural change, but it is not the common pattern.

Prioritising problems, sharing the overall plan and proceeding in a stepwise fashion

Strategies are built up from tactics. Individual interventions are the component parts that form a larger and logical strategy towards an overall treatment goal. Treatment is best planned in stages, with as few interventions being introduced simultaneously as possible. This allows evaluation of the outcome of the one intervention before deciding whether the next is necessary. Working out priorities with the patient helps to form an outline of a sequence of interventions that will plausibly improve things. Certain problems demand immediate attention because nothing else is likely to help until they are under control, as was the case with Mr Kennedy's heavy drinking. Sometimes it is important to help the patient to tackle a pressing practical problem first because it is weighing so heavily upon them, for example, debt management or welfare benefit entitlements. Sometimes achieving symptomatic improvement is the most prominent priority, as is often the case where someone is acutely psychotic or severely anxious.

There are only two real rules here. Firstly, there is no point in prioritising a problem that is unlikely to be amenable to change. If a young man has been smoking a lot of cannabis for several years, and he has built a social life around cannabis smoking, he is unlikely to stop just because a middle-aged, middle-class professional says so. Although chronic cannabis intoxication can exacerbate psychosis, anxiety and depression, delaying symptomatic treatment until it is under control is rarely successful. Secondly, tackling problems that have a strong bearing on risk should only be delayed with caution. For example, it may be the case that risk is reduced by forming a good therapeutic relationship with the patient, but this takes time. It may be perfectly possible to form a therapeutic alliance with a jealous deluded man. However, the fact that warning his partner that she is at risk of violence may make it more difficult to work with him does not justify delaying or failing to make the warning.

Initially, the overall plan may not be very detailed, but the likely general pattern of treatment usually is clear. In the case of Mr Kennedy, it was uncertain exactly how much treatment he was likely to need, but it was still possible to set out an overall plan. It is particularly useful for the psychiatrist to make it clear how the sequence of interventions fits together, because the patient is more likely to do as the professional suggests if the plan makes sense to them.

It is not always the case that the overall likely pattern is clear at the outset. Sometimes you just have to take the obvious and sensible first step, see what happens, and then decide what to do next. This is, in itself, a treatment plan, and the uncertainty over next steps can be shared. This would apply in many situations where the patient is encountered for the first time in the context of an emergency, and it is evident that he needs hospitalisation. It is unusual under these circumstances to have sufficient information to make a detailed long-term plan, but people are often reassured by the fact that you tell them that there will be a long-term plan involving help outside of the hospital setting, and that they will be involved in planning their longer term treatment.

Anticipating and evaluating setbacks, and deciding whether to change the plan

Psychiatric treatment can proceed very smoothly, and sometimes things go far better than you expected. Mostly, however, there are setbacks along the way. We quite regularly find ourselves wondering if we are doing something seriously wrong, because the patient is not improving. Sometimes we start to worry that we are actually making the patient worse. Most of the time, a well thought-through strategy does eventually work, but what makes life difficult is the fact that sometimes it turns out that we *are* doing something wrong or we *are* making the patient worse not better. This is an ambiguity that has to be managed, because setbacks are one of the main factors that can derail treatment strategies and lead the clinician back to a reactive approach, with attendant polypharmacy, loss of direction and worse. Box 4.1 sets out some of the indicators that treatment is failing. We do not suggest that these things can always be avoided. However, if you look out for the accumulation of these indicators, you are likely to recognise that things are going wrong sooner rather than later, creating an opportunity to reconsider the overall strategy.

Box 4.1 Ten incrementally ominous signs that treatment is failing

1. The patient is on more than two psychotropic medications.
2. There are frequent changes of medication.
3. Discussion in consultations is focussed on the merits of different medications and subtle variations in symptoms. There is little discussion of the patient's daily activities, the stresses in their life and their plans for the future.
4. There is a pattern of increasingly frequent appointments. You feel a little apprehensive about suggesting longer gaps between appointments.
5. Either you or the patient expresses the belief that you will eventually get the medication right (the 'magic cocktail' myth).
6. The diagnosis is adjusted to conform to responses to medication.
7. You suggest adding a mood stabilising anticonvulsant, despite the fact that the patient does not suffer from bipolar affective disorder.
8. You start to wonder if the patient was abused in childhood, despite the complete absence of any such history from the patient.
9. The patient tells you that you are the only person he has to talk to.
10. You explore the Internet to investigate novel treatment technologies involving, for example, magnets and flashing lights.

Life goes on remorselessly during psychiatric treatment, and all lives have ups and downs. Everyone tends to feel bad in the face of the vagaries of fortune. For people with mental illnesses, problems in their lives can make them feel bad in the same way as anyone else, but they can also lead to a worsening of symptoms. This is one of a number of reasons why it is unusual for patients to be a bit better at each consecutive interview until they eventually come and say that they are back to their old selves. Just because the patient is not feeling so good at a particular interview does not necessarily mean that treatment is not working. The question is rather, is there an overall trajectory of improvement and is the improvement occurring at a pace and to the extent that one would expect, taking into account the various contextual factors bearing upon the patient? This is something that has to be worked out by the patient and the professional together, sometimes with the help of the patient's family, who are often in a better position than anyone else to recognise how things are proceeding.

The next problem is 'I'm feeling better but...' The 'but' is commonly either a side effect ('Since I've been on fluoxetine I'm a lot better but I can't get an orgasm and it's affecting my relationship') or a symptom that is slow to improve ('I'm feeling a lot better but I still can't sleep'). It is not the case that it is necessarily wrong to change medications under these circumstances. If there is to be an alteration in medication it is better to change from one drug to another than to add drugs (such as night sedation). However, all drugs have side effects, and it is possible to lose one side effect only to gain a worse one (followed by another change). The doctor and the patient need to think about the cost–benefit equation ('What is the overall balance of effects here'), bearing in mind factors such as the likely length of time that the patient will need to take the drug and therefore have to put up with the side effects. Furthermore, symptoms tend to improve at different tempos, and sometimes it is best to wait for a symptom to resolve.

A strategic approach to treatment does not dictate rigid adherence to an initial plan. One of the patterns of behaviour that can lead to mental health problems arises where people have a maladaptive way of coping with distress (for example, through avoidance, or self-harm or clinging dependency) which eventually starts to fail (for example, because avoidance tends to lead to more anxiety, or because self-harm or clinging dependency starts to exasperate other people). Instead of changing their behaviour, they escalate a strategy which has already failed, and the situation progressively deteriorates. This can be mirrored by psychiatrists who fail to recognise that a treatment is failing strategically, and try to bolster the potency of an approach that is not working. It would seem self-evident that, if a patient is still depressed despite taking a combination of two antidepressants, adding a further drug is unlikely to do the trick. Unfortunately, it is not difficult to find yourself presiding over this kind of disorganised treatment. The patient gains some protection from this if the clinician, faced with a setback or a lack of expected response, routinely asks himself 'Is the strategy failing, or is it only partly successful?' and 'How long should I allow things to go along like this before I change strategy?'

To return to Mr Kennedy, the overall treatment strategy can accommodate quite a range of setbacks without major modification. He might struggle to stop drinking, in which case specialist alcohol services can be involved without bringing treatment of his underlying depression to a halt. On the other hand, he might stop drinking, start taking an antidepressant at a standard dose, experience some improvement in his mood, but still complain that he is waking early with pessimistic thoughts about the future. This might mean that his marital problems are unchanged and that this is impeding his recovery, in which case a marital intervention might be necessary. It might reflect a partial response to antidepressants, in which case the dose may need adjustment. However, if depressive symptoms persist despite a resolution of most of the apparent difficulties in his life, it would be important for Dr Jackson to consider the possibility that he missed something at the beginning, such as an undisclosed affair or hypothyroidism.

Sometimes it is helpful to predict setbacks, because they are likely and people cope better with them if they know that they do not mean that everything is going to go back to square one. Predicting that symptoms will sometimes return is an intrinsic part of cognitive and behavioural treatments for anxiety disorders. These treatments tend to emphasise the patient's ability to control symptoms rather than attempting to completely abolish them. This emphasis is useful in the management of a range of other symptoms, including residual hallucinations due to chronic schizophrenia.

Maintaining realistic therapeutic optimism

Instillation of hope is widely regarded as a key therapeutic factor in all types of mental health work, so it is dispiriting to find that one of the more consistent complaints of the service user movement is that psychiatry has historically tended to convey an expectation that recovery is not possible. As we discussed in Chapter 3, recovery is about regaining autonomy and a sense of well being. It does not rest upon an unrealistic therapeutic heroism. Indeed, the unrealistic expectation that symptoms, or a vulnerability to relapse, can be abolished is an impediment to recovery. Recovery often means learning to manage one's symptoms and vulnerabilities. Attempts to abolish symptoms that have persisted for decades, such as hallucinations or chronic anxiety, are rarely effective. In the long run, such a treatment objective is bound to undermine hope. On the other hand, recognising that these things are likely to persist, but that there may be ways of managing them that may lead to improvements in the person's life can be surprisingly liberating.

Therapeutic heroism can develop unnoticed within a team until it suddenly causes a problem. If one team member is quietly working towards unrealisable goals, this can derail the effectiveness of the whole team intervention. This can arise during the placement of a particularly enthusiastic but inexperienced learner, who starts working heroically and then moves on before the consequences become apparent. Politically incorrect psychiatrists call this 'the curse of the student social worker', though it could equally well be labelled 'the curse of the locum psychiatrist'. Similar problems can arise if you plough on with treatment after significant improvement in the belief that your work is not done until the patient's life 'comes right'. Therapeutic optimism frequently involves the recognition that the mental health professional's role in facilitating recovery has limitations, and that other processes are important as well.

Recognising when enough has been achieved

It follows from this that the termination of treatment needs to be well timed. This can mean recognising that there are unlikely to be further gains from intervention. Some times, when the person's life is on a clear trajectory of improvement, it is best to discharge them relatively early, before 'full' recovery. If patients know that they can return if things go wrong, the professional's confidence in their ability to resolve problems for themselves, demonstrated by 'letting them get on with it', can be an important therapeutic statement. This is not to condone half completed treatment plans and the abandonment of patients at the drop of a hat. The judgement as to when enough is enough has to be made by the patient and professional together, and it can take some time to properly work such decisions through. It usually involves gradually handing responsibility for well being back to the patient in an explicit way.

Recording strategic plans

It can be difficult to record strategic plans. They can be complicated, and writing them out longhand is time consuming. They are sometimes formulated in meetings with patients, or in team meetings, and hence they are lost in routine paperwork. Earlier in our careers, we tended to hold strategic plans in our heads, and shared them through discussions with patients. This was not a good idea. Explicit plans are essential in team working, and if a plan is not explicit, it is difficult for another team member to pick up the threads if you are off sick or change jobs. We strongly recommend that strategic plans are recorded in case notes as they develop, and we find that this is best achieved by dictating notes after every interview (wherever it occurs) and after every formal team discussion. This does throw some pressure on secretarial staff, but there are overwhelming advantages in having an accessible and clear record of the rationale behind treatment plans, and the reasons for changes as they occur. We find it much easier to do this using a voice recorder than by writing longhand. Modern computer systems allow such typed notes to be available when they are needed, for example, to staff who assess patients in out-of-hours emergencies.

Main points in this chapter

1. Successful treatment rests on a good understanding of the contextual factors that affect the patient's mental well being and on getting alongside them therapeutically.
2. Treatment objectives should be explicit and formulated in partnership with the patient and his family.
3. Interventions should be prioritised and sequenced. Psychiatrists have to resist the temptation to do too much too soon.
4. Risk management should be, as far as possible, a joint task of professionals and patients.
5. All lives have ups and downs, and this has to be borne in mind in deciding if a treatment strategy is failing.
6. Many of the factors leading to recovery belong to patients, not mental health professionals. Maintaining realistic optimism is a therapeutic task that can be undermined, rather than supported, by trying to pursue treatment until the patient is 'properly' better.
7. Strategic plans need to be clearly recorded in such a way that they are available to other team members.

Part II – The context and location of treatment

In the assessment of people suffering from mental illness, understanding the context of the problem (which is to say the patient's personality, life history and current circumstances) is of crucial importance. The context of treatment is similarly of critical importance in making it effective.

Psychiatric treatment is carried out by teams of varying size. Chapters 5 and 6 deal with a range of issues concerning teams and team working.

Although admission to hospital and treatment under duress are to be avoided if at all possible, they are bound to happen sometimes. Chapters 7, 8 and 9 address neglected issues of the location of care and the use of legal compulsion.

Psychiatric treatment occurs in a context of social policy and public attitudes, both of which have a tangible impact on the type of care offered and the relationship between clinicians and service users. These issues are discussed in Chapter 10.

5 Teams

Who is a part of the team?

All psychiatrists work in teams, large or small. Most UK psychiatrists have grown up working in large teams, and the intrinsic complexity of these teams tends to go unnoticed because of familiarity. However, anyone who has struggled to explain the workings of a Community Mental Health Team (CMHT) to a bewildered medical student quickly realises that there is nothing straightforward about teamwork in psychiatry.

One of us is a member of a CMHT that comprises nineteen people, all based in a building within the community it serves. There is office space for members of other teams, and there are close working relationships with teams based elsewhere. Box 5.1 sets out the membership of these three concentric circles of staff and specialist teams. It takes a lot of effort and organisation, together with a sophisticated understanding of systems and team dynamics, to ensure that such a complex configuration of professionals functions smoothly and appropriately. Fortunately the primary responsibility for this rarely lies with the psychiatrist.

Many psychiatrists, for example, in the UK private sector and office-based practitioners in North America, work in much smaller teams (sometimes just the psychiatrist and a secretary/receptionist). We would suggest that attention to teamwork is no less important in these very small teams than in larger ones. Indeed, the problems in a large team caused by a dysfunctional team member pale into insignificance compared to the problems caused by a bad working relationship between an isolated psychiatrist and his secretary.

Teams can only function optimally if everyone does their job well. Disorganised clerical staff and maintenance workers can bring a team to a standstill just as easily as a disorganised psychiatrist. From the point of view of team functioning, social status is irrelevant. Everyone is important. Human beings have a strong tendency to work well if they are acknowledged as people and if they know that their work is valued. Secretaries, reception staff and records clerks have pivotal roles. They are privy to a great deal of confidential information, and they have to decide what to do in the face of a wide variety of unexpected circumstances. Not only do they need to be well organised; they can only carry out their work effectively if they understand both their own role and the purpose and underlying values of the whole team. This understanding cannot emerge spontaneously. Taking care to help them to understand mental health and the reasons for doing things in a particular way makes an enormous difference to their job satisfaction and occupational functioning.

Box 5.1 Team membership

Core membership of CMHT:
- Community mental health nurses
- Social workers
- Secretaries, receptionists and records clerks
- Occupational therapists
- Psychiatrists
- Support workers
- Psychologist
- Team manager

Teams with office space in same building:
- Assertive Outreach Team
- Primary Care Liaison Team
- Substance Dependency Team

Teams with a close working relationship with CMHT:
- Inpatient team
- Social Care Day Services
- Crisis Resolution and Home Treatment Team
- Acute Hospital Liaison Team
- General Practices
- Voluntary Sector Mental Health Services

The best piece of advice we ever give our trainees is *don't fall out with the secretary.* If you do, the patients may or may not suffer, but you certainly will. We suggest that the use of possessive pronouns with regard to team members is best avoided, e.g. '*the* secretary' and '*the* community mental health nurse', not '*my*' or '*your*'. This does not reflect a pedantic attachment to political correctness. The use of possessive pronouns in this context reveals an unhealthy attitude to the relationship between a psychiatrist and the rest of the team. Possession is a quality in human relationships which is normally associated with either intimacy or slavery, neither of which is at all helpful in effective teamwork.

Mental health practice involves collaboration between different teams and different agencies. This means that it is not always clear exactly who is in the team and who is outside of it. Like all social configurations, mental health teams need boundaries in order to maintain their stability and to function appropriately. A key boundary concerns membership, which means that there must be clarity over the difference between those who are team members and those who are close colleagues working outside of the team. Without this, confidences can be unwittingly broken and responsibility can be diffused. To further complicate matters, in the UK it is common for professionals within the team to be employed by different organisations, for example National Health Service Trusts and local authority Social Service departments.

As a rule of thumb, a mental health team exists where a group of people works to a common goal as (or under the supervision of) trained mental health professionals. A team can only be said to exist if its members share an office or a working base that allows them face-to-face communication both formally and, just as importantly, informally in the course of the working week. A dispersed group of professionals may be called a team, but there can be no meaningful teamwork unless individuals meet together on a very regular basis. The culture of some professions, notably clinical psychology, has a strong emphasis on working individually with patients. This can make it difficult for them to participate in teamwork. Even when they are based in the same place as everyone else, they may function essentially separately and autonomously. (Where psychologists participate as full team members, they are absolutely invaluable. We are not criticising a more individual style of intervention, but under these circumstances they cannot be regarded as part of the team.)

Clarity over the location and membership of the team is especially important in providing robust channels of communication in emergencies and in providing reliable backup and cover. If communication and backup depends upon people who are not really team members, these systems are vulnerable to failure when they are most needed. In community teams it is absolutely essential that someone at the team base knows where every member of the team is meant to be (and where they actually are if this is likely to be different) at all times. This is necessary for personal safety, but it is also important to team functioning, because sometimes the specific expertise of individuals is needed at short notice.

Who does the team belong to?

Experience is an invaluable guide to improving practice, provided you retain a capacity for reflection and a degree of self-awareness. Unfortunately, some of the things you learn are not especially palatable, particularly when they contradict cherished beliefs about yourself and your profession. One of the hardest lessons we have had to learn has been that, out of all of the disciplines that work in mental health, psychiatrists have the greatest ability to disrupt and undermine good teamwork. Harder still has been the realisation that we have sometimes been personally culpable of this. Box 5.2 contains a true story.

Naturally enough, we do not think that psychiatrists disrupt teams because they are unusually narcissistic or insensitive people (though we may be mistaken in this belief). The problem with doctors is their special status. Doctors often look back wistfully to a time before there were litigious ex-patients, complaints procedures, ever more demanding reaccreditation procedures, serious untoward incident inquiries and clinical guidelines. Internationally there is a mood within the medical profession that the good times have long passed. Doctors these days seem to feel battered, maligned and misunderstood. Whilst there is no doubt that unquestioning acquiescence to medical opinion is disappearing, an objective appraisal suggests that this has had little effect on the social status of doctors. They are well paid and opinion polls suggest that they

Box 5.2 The return of the king

Dr Bob was a consultant psychiatrist with a good reputation as a skilled clinician. He was proud of the quality of care that the CMHT offered in a tough inner-city area. He had a forceful and colourful personality, which had a significant impact on the team culture. Team members either enjoyed working with him, or disliked the working atmosphere and left.

Dr Bob was also a medical manager. He was offered a one-year secondment in order to gain experience at a more senior managerial level. He did not want to leave his team, because he enjoyed his clinical work and he feared that they would struggle without him. However, he accepted the secondment in the belief that no one is indispensable and that, in the end, it would be good for him and the team.

At the end of the year, Dr Bob returned to his regular job. He knew that there had been problems in his absence with some unsatisfactory locum psychiatrists. He expected the team to be relieved and pleased at his return.

On his first day back, the community mental health nurses and the secretary took him to a room 'for a chat'. They explained that they had completely reorganised the way that the team worked. The team manager said 'We won't tolerate your disorgan-isation again. If you mess things up and everything goes back to how it was before, we're leaving'. The others all nodded and said 'Yes, we will all leave'.

Dr Bob felt a little crushed. All he could do was to go along with their new systems and see how things worked out. At first the changes seemed mainly restrictive. He was not allowed to accept referrals without discussion with the rest of the team. He was only allowed to see patients alone if there was a specific reason for him to do so. He was expected to dictate letters on the same day that he saw the patient. He was expected to do some paperwork every day. Before very long it became obvious that his work load was substantially less than it had been. He spent more time with patients, and his work was more focussed. He relinquished responsibility for overall team working to the team manager. He was calmer and less stressed, and so was the rest of the team.

The most difficult aspect of the situation was that he had to acknowledge that the team was working much more effectively. Their capacity to deal with emergen-cies was much improved. Routine reviews still happened regularly, but they were less frequent and were a smaller part of the team's overall workload. He reluctantly recognised that his role in the team and his working practices had been a major problem for everyone in the past.

are highly trusted professionals. It seems unlikely to us that this is going to change. In the Soviet Union there was a concerted effort to remake the medical profession. Doctors were paid less than the national average salary, but they frequently received payment in kind from their patients. Their primary responsibility was to the state, not to the individual patient, but they were generally trusted and continued to enjoy a special social status. It would seem that doctors and kudos cannot be easily separated.

Box 5.3 Eleven tips for psychiatrists who want to disrupt their team

1. Maintain an office base separate from the rest of the team, preferably several miles away.
2. Cultivate poor time keeping and do not apologise for it. Expect the rest of the team to accept persistent lateness.
3. Allow paperwork to fall behind. There should be a good delay between seeing patients and dictating letters, and between them being typed and being signed. Do not correct typing errors.
4. Keep case notes locked in your office, or better still, in your briefcase.
5. Make major decisions outside of meetings and multidisciplinary reviews.
6. Make undertakings that affect team members without consulting them. This is particularly potent where the undertaking is made to another doctor. Indeed, the hidden hand of the freemasonry of medicine is a device that can cause mischief in a wide variety of circumstances.
7. Avoid fully explaining your decisions to patients and other team members.
8. Expect your concerns and preoccupations to be given priority as a natural right.
9. Insist that team members should continue to see patients when they feel that this is unnecessary or inappropriate.
10. Develop idiosyncratic treatment approaches that have a weak or non-existent evidence base.
11. Regularly remind the team of the sacred and unique bond between doctor and patient.

Social status and authority, if deployed judiciously, can be useful in persuading people to accept unpalatable but good advice. It is vexing that some patients reject advice from non-medical professionals, only to act on the same advice when it comes from the doctor. Although paternalism is outmoded and has few apologists, nearly all teams use the psychiatrist as heavy artillery from time to time, because it works. Unfortunately it is exactly this inequity of authority and influence that can make psychiatrists so disruptive. The fact that one team member's opinion is likely to carry greater weight than everyone else's distorts decision making. Opinions should be taken seriously because they are well informed, rational and reasonable, not because of the professional's job title. There are some adverse effects of inequities in authority when the psychiatrist is liked, respected and has sound judgement. There are more serious consequences where other team members struggle to contain the impact of a psychiatrist's poor judgement. Under these circumstances, authority tends to be wielded as a blunt weapon, because the psychiatrist will not be liked or trusted by the team.

Psychiatrists tend to work best in teams when they accept that they are not in charge, and that their time and expertise is a team resource. It is probably inevitable that psychiatrists carry the greatest authority in clinical matters, but having authority and trying to control everything are very different. A key issue is the control of referrals and their allocation within the team, as this has a significant impact on a range of other team functions.

It is generally best if control of referrals into the team is the responsibility of a team manager, who also has to ensure that each team member's case mix and case load is appropriate. If control of referrals rests with a consultant psychiatrist, as has traditionally been the case in the UK, then de facto control of the overall case load lies with him. Psychiatrists rarely have the expertise to manage the allocation and turnover of patients within the team. It is almost inevitable under these circumstances that the psychiatrist exerts increasing pressure on the rest of the team to take on cases and discourages discharges. He becomes the default professional who sees patients if the team is working at or over capacity. In the absence of a proper system to manage work load, other team members tend to establish systems to avoid taking on more cases. The outcome is a stressed and overworked psychiatrist, an unhappy team and serious problems in ensuring that patients have access to timely multidisciplinary care. No matter what the stated philosophy of the team, parallel working and traditional clinics, with all their faults (see Chapters 6 and 9), are the only ways that a team can function under these conditions.

On the other hand, a team manager who has control over the processing and allocation of referrals is in a much better position to optimally deploy the totality of team time. Provided the team manager recognises the pitfalls of allowing the psychiatrist to be the default professional, the outcome is more efficient, and life is more pleasant for everyone. This does not imply that psychiatrists should have no role in the triage of referrals or in their assessment. Medical input is an intrinsic component of all multidisciplinary processes. It is the primacy of the medical role that is questionable. Where the psychiatrist is a team resource, rather than vice versa, it is much easier to control his work load and to focus his expertise on those situations where it is most needed.

There are a variety of routine team meetings that focus on day-to-day clinical decision making, including 'ward rounds' (an oddly archaic term that shows little sign of dying out), referral meetings, Care Programme Approach reviews and multidisciplinary team meetings (the UK term for the main CMHT meeting of the week). Although the medical component of these meetings is intrinsically important, chairmanship is best held by someone other than the psychiatrist, usually the team manager. There is both a practical and a symbolic importance in ensuring that the meeting belongs to, and solves problems for, the whole team. This is not guaranteed by non-medical chairmanship, but it helps. Similarly, the location of meetings should be decided primarily by convenience to, in order of priority, the patient and their family, the team and the doctor.

Leadership

Even in the most hierarchical of social structures, such as the armed forces, leadership is a complex phenomenon. Although power can be attached to a professional role or job description, leadership cannot. Although certain professional roles, both managerial and clinical, carry an expectation of leadership, it does not happen automatically.

Individuals acquire leadership by one of two routes. Ideally, it is granted by the larger group because an individual has competence and credibility. They lead because they command general respect. Leadership can also be seized through intimidation and bullying. Leadership dysfunction within teams can arise in a number of different ways. Sometimes the senior role in the team is held by someone who fails to command respect. Sometimes, although respected, they are unwilling or unable to use leadership constructively. In either case this creates a leadership vacuum. Under these circumstances, someone else is likely to emerge as the leader of the team, and this may or may not be an individual who uses his influence in a constructive way. Even where there is a strong leader, a bullying team member can create a dual leadership structure, where team members are torn between the conflicting expectations of a legitimate leader who is respected and an illegitimate leader who is feared.

Needless to say, a doctor may acquire leadership by either route, but one cannot assume that they are the most appropriate or the inevitable leader of the team just because of their job title and qualifications. Whether they take the leadership role or not, they need *clinical authority* as an essential personal characteristic. Senior professionals of all disciplines need this. Clinical authority arises where it is clear that you have good clinical skills, a good knowledge base and sound judgement. Clinical authority is enhanced by an evident awareness of the extent and limitations of one's expertise, which means having respect for the fact that other disciplines have a different and valid perspective.

Both clinical authority and clinical leadership are different from managerial authority, which can only rest with a line manager. It is not uncommon for there to be multiple line managerial relationships within a team. For example, doctors frequently work alongside a team manager who is not strictly speaking their line manager. These multiple threads of managerial authority, clinical authority and clinical leadership create ample opportunity for confusion.

Effective teams

Although teams can be organised in a number of different ways, functional teamwork tends to follow a few themes. Dysfunctional teamwork, on the other hand, is polymorphous. There are a lot of different ways in which it can all go wrong. Some of the common features of functional teams include:

- There is a clear leader. Those other individuals who carry managerial or clinical authority work to support the clinical leader and avoid creating ambiguity as to who is in charge.
- Debate is encouraged, and dissent is tolerated. Differences are resolved in team meetings, rather than through impromptu discussions. Such debates are allowed to continue long enough for a way to be found to accommodate differences of opinion. This may mean agreeing to a course of action that you do not believe will work on the understanding that, if it does indeed fail, the alternative will then prevail.
- Team members have clarity over their roles and responsibilities. In particular, people do not assume that someone else will resolve problems; they make sure that

the appropriate person is aware of a problem and that something is being done about it.

- Deviant behaviour by team members is recognised and dealt with. Such behaviour can range from judgemental attitudes and breaches of therapeutic boundaries through to frank bullying or neglect of professional responsibilities. In functional teams, such problems are resolved by a line manager or clinical supervisor. The staff member is clearly warned that his behaviour is unacceptable at an early stage. Responses follow a timely and logical progression from the low key and informal to the formal and disciplinary according to whether things improve. Records are kept. There is continued monitoring of the situation because, whilst everyone likes to hope that these problems will go away, they are often recurrent.

- The team has fun together. This is always important for team cohesion. It may mean that the team meets for social gatherings, but these can sometimes prove to be destructive. Not everyone wants to socialise with work colleagues, and the expectation that they should do so can be intrusive. Alcohol can encourage people to behave in ways that permanently affect working relationships. Finding a place for humour and playfulness within the team is probably more reliable than social events, because work is enjoyable when there is some fun day by day. However, this requires an awareness of the essential seriousness of the job. Where fun and work are in conflict, work must always prevail.

- The team's found assets are used and developed. These are the personal interests and skills of individual team members. Encouraging professionals to develop particular interests and skills expands the team's expertise. It does tend to mean that team members move on through promotion, but this encourages good staff members to come and work with the team, because they have a reasonable expectation of professional development.

Generic teams or specialist teams?

Psychiatry can be organised primarily through genericism (whereby small numbers of large teams try to help people with a broad range of problems) and specialism (whereby a larger number of small teams each try to help people with a narrow range of problems). In the UK, psychiatry was traditionally hospital based and generic. In the 1960s and 1970s a pattern of hospital-based specialisation started, which led to the emergence of distinct sub-specialities such as forensic psychiatry, old age psychiatry, rehabilitation psychiatry and so forth, leaving a residual generic service for adults of working age. In the 1980s, community psychiatry developed out of general adult psychiatry, with the formation of generic CMHTs. Since the late 1990s there has been another, more rapid, wave of sub-specialisation as a matter of national policy. To a varying extent in different locations, CMHTs have relinquished some of their work to crisis resolution and home treatment teams, assertive outreach teams, continuing care teams, early intervention teams and primary care liaison teams.

It is futile to take a position as to whether genericism or specialism is preferable. It is difficult to evaluate the effectiveness of specific patterns of service delivery,

---

Box 5.4 Some features of generic and specialist teams

Generic teams:

- Offer general services to a locality, so there can be no doubt over who should provide a service.
- Can develop close working relationships with other local agencies, particularly primary care.
- Can be based within the community they serve.
- Are easily able to offer integrated care and continuity of care.
- May allow individual team members to develop special interests and areas of particular expertise.
- Are easily overwhelmed by pressure of work, because they must offer both routine and emergency care.
- May only manage to offer lowest common denominator care, owing to lack of specific expertise.
- Tend to look like a woolly idea on paper but can work very well.

Specialist teams:

- Are able to work within specific models that can be evaluated.
- Develop specific skills within the whole team.
- Have a clear focus.
- Can create a bewildering array of services.
- Can create 'criteria gaps' whereby some people with unusual problems cannot access any service.
- Create multiple interfaces, with attendant problems as patients cross these interfaces.
- Cover large areas and therefore are not truly local.
- Have to involve other teams when problems arise beyond their specific remit.
- Tend to look very logical on paper, but can work very badly.

---

as is illustrated by the ambiguous evidence regarding assertive outreach in the UK (Killaspy *et al.*, 2006). It is essentially impossible to empirically evaluate the strengths and weaknesses of total systems of care. However, genericism and specialism have distinct advantages and pitfalls.

At the present time we have a mixture of more specialist teams and more generic teams. This may or may not be the best of both worlds. The trend to specialisation is evident throughout the developed world, and it has a momentum that would be hard to stop. Some hold the view that CMHTs are outmoded, and that they will before long disappear. We believe that generic CMHTs for people with serious mental illness have major advantages, and that these should not be lost. Continuity of care, the ability to really understand a local community and to develop close working relationships with primary care are features of CMHT working that cannot be replicated by specialist teams. We cannot point to unequivocal empirical evidence that they are important. However, we believe that these are major strengths that allow good quality care to be provided to people suffering from acute psychosis in their own homes. There is a danger that evidence supporting this belief will only become available when the consequences of abolishing genericism have become evident.

CMHTs can only function if there is a capability within the team to provide help with substance misuse problems, to carry out some psychological therapies (especially CBT) and to work to a truly biopsychosocial model. However, there is also a need for clarity as to the team's limitations. Some problems will be beyond the expertise of the very best of CMHTs. Although the need for specialist involvement may become evident because the patient does not get better, sometimes it is evident from the outset that a problem is likely to require specialist help. There is often a temptation to have a go yourself before making a referral (and sometimes funding bodies demand this). This can be a mistake. An inexpert attempt to deploy a treatment can foreclose the possibility of more expert intervention. For example, obsessive-compulsive disorder may respond to behavioural therapies or CBT, but they rarely work when deployed by an untrained or unsupervised therapist. If some parts of these therapies are used and fail, it is very difficult for an expert to have a second try (not least because the patient is likely to feel 'I've tried this before and it failed'). Individuals and whole teams need to be aware of the scope and limitations of their own skills.

Seeking advice from outside of the team

It can be helpful to involve specialist teams when dealing with specific problems that demand particular expertise, for example, from forensic psychiatry or learning disability teams. If the involvement of specialist teams from time to time is a necessary part of CMHT working, second opinions are much more difficult and ambiguous. Patients and their families sometimes want a second opinion on diagnosis or treatment options, and this is entirely legitimate. However, the majority of second opinions are initiated by the psychiatrist.

Experienced and self-confident psychiatrists regularly talk difficult clinical situations over with their colleagues. They contact experts for advice when they start to feel stuck. Most will have at least one relationship with a colleague that amounts to a co-supervision. It is not that they expect their colleague to solve problems for them. The process of reflection and discussion helps to clarify thinking, tests the robustness of one's hypotheses about situations, and thus helps to find ways forward. In our experience, these two processes help to resolve most situations that would otherwise lead to a request for a second opinion.

The problem with second opinions is that they are often unproductive. There is certainly no point in asking for a second opinion unless you are prepared to act on the recommendations that you are given. A second opinion that you will only act on if it confirms your thinking and will ignore if it does not is a complete waste of time. When one has exhausted the team's capacity to deal with a problem, referral to a tertiary centre for treatment can be helpful. However, tertiary centres are often a long way away, and the local service may be left to manage the overall situation week by week in between appointments with the experts. This leads to dual management and ambiguity as to whether plans should be altered in the face of new developments in the situation. Tertiary centres are at a serious disadvantage when asked to give just a second opinion and advice on treatment. They can only carry out a snapshot assessment. The advice they give is often algorithmic, and as such only tells you what you already know. This tends to confirm your sense that the situation is irresolvable. Sometimes they give advice to do what they would do, which is usually impossible to implement, because you do not have their facilities or expertise to carry out special treatment regimes.

Second opinions from local colleagues can be helpful, but after a few years in post you get to know your colleagues well, and you can soon predict what they are likely to say. As a consequence, such second opinions may not solve problems. There are some situations, usually involving risk, where you need to demonstrate that you have ensured that your judgement is sound and that your plan is appropriate. Asking for a colleague's opinion is then important and legitimate. The procedure is, however, essentially defensive and problem solving is not the objective.

Main points in this chapter

1. Do not fall out with the secretary.
2. Teams only exist when they routinely meet together, formally and informally, in the course of the working week.
3. Psychiatrists work best where they are a resource for the team rather than vice versa.
4. Psychiatrists may find that they are the de facto leader of the team. However, it is not inevitable, nor necessarily desirable, that leadership should rest with them.
5. Advice and reflection with colleagues is helpful when struggling with difficult problems. Second opinions are rarely helpful, except as a defensive manoeuvre.

6   Teamwork

The medical and nursing professions have a reciprocal dependency. Neither discipline could have a meaningful existence without the other. However, each has a distinctive culture, and one of the differences between them concerns their attitude to team working. Nurse training and culture tend to generate professionals who are most comfortable as members of teams. Consequently, nurses can find professional autonomy difficult. Medical training and culture tend to generate professionals who are most comfortable as individualistic decision makers. Doctors can find teamwork difficult to understand, because they tend to think that they should be unambiguously in charge. Psychiatrists are no exception, and they can struggle to be good team players.

Successful teamwork depends on qualities of the team and on individual skills. Effective teams are greater than the sum of their parts. Team members are interdependent in their roles, which means that communication between them has to be effective and continuous. Those team members who are in a position of leadership or authority have to manage the tension between non-hierarchical multidisciplinary working and the occasional need to override consensus (for example, when individual expertise indicates that some factor is more significant than other team members appreciate). Perhaps the single most important personal attribute of good team players is that they are comfortable in their professional roles, which is to say both self-confident and accepting of their limitations. Psychiatrists who lack these qualities either prevaricate and lose credibility or become authoritarian and defensive, neither of which is compatible with effective teamwork.

Joint working

Teams can work together in a wide variety of ways. In CMHTs the key to effective teamwork is that professionals from different disciplines see patients together on a regular basis. Individual work is conducted to achieve specific objectives, but the backbone of team activity is joint work. The alternative to joint working is parallel working. Parallel working was the dominant model of teamwork in UK mental health practice for many years. It has two main drawbacks. As different professionals meet with patients alone and on separate occasions, it is hard to integrate interventions into an overall strategic plan. Decisions tend to occur without reference to other professionals' observations and opinions. This invites the development of separate or parallel treatment plans and eventual incoherence of treatment. The other main drawback is the risk that a team member develops a special and exclusive relationship with the patient. This makes it very difficult for other team members to work effectively. At worst it can be the first step along the road to a breach of boundaries and an abusive therapeutic relationship. Box 6.1 gives an example of how this can occur.

Box 6.1 A special relationship

Diane was a thirty-one-year-old woman with a twelve-year history of bipolar affective disorder. She had had a difficult childhood with periods in local authority care and repeated exclusion from school. As an adult she remained impulsive. She easily resorted to verbal aggression in the face of trivial frustrations. She found authority figures hard to tolerate, and she tended to be truculent in her dealings with mental health professionals. When manic she was unpleasant, aggressive and difficult to manage. She had a certain notoriety amongst the mental health services, and she fell out with a succession of community mental health nurses.

Ann was a thirty-year-old mental health nurse who had recently returned to full-time work after having two children. She had been an inpatient nurse, but the needs of her young family had dictated a change to the more regular hours in community nursing. She had nursed Diane during acute manic episodes, and she felt some apprehension when she found that she was now on her case load in the community. However, Diane was pleased. During the recovery phase of manic episodes she had often chatted to Ann on the ward, and she liked her. Ann was surprised to find that Diane was more amenable than she had expected. She was willing to give her extra time as their relationship strengthened. Diane soon told Ann that she was the best nurse that she had met and that if only other staff had treated her like this her relationship with the service would not have been so turbulent. Diane still ranted and raved about minor problems, but Ann found that, if she stayed calm, Diane's anger passed, and she could reason with her to find more productive ways of dealing with problems. They had a special relationship.

Ann came to feel that it was best if other staff did not see Diane when she was absent from work. She feared that old patterns of interaction would return, and that the ground she had gained would be lost. Diane tended to find doctors provocative, and Ann would cancel review meetings if Diane was in a bad mood. She encouraged Diane to let her do the talking when meetings did occur.

Everything went wrong when Ann fell pregnant again. As maternity leave approached, Diane became increasingly angry at being abandoned, and she refused to co-operate with her replacement. Soon after Ann's leave started, Diane stopped her medication and would not open the door when mental health professionals called. There was no return to her earlier position of sullen co-operation under duress. Now she was hostile and rejecting of services, and she rapidly relapsed into acute mania. There was an unseemly and traumatic drama at the house when she was compulsorily taken to hospital. The police smashed down the door, and dragged her to the ambulance. She arrived at the hospital in handcuffs.

The trouble with special relationships is that they are also exclusive relationships.

We have described the process of conducting a joint interview elsewhere (Poole & Higgo, 2006). A few points are worth reiterating here. Each joint interview should have a specified purpose, explicitly agreed between the professionals beforehand. These might include review of medication, routine review of care plan (in which case there is a low expectation that the interview will lead to change), diagnostic interview, interview to give information to patient and family, review of treatment options in anticipation of planned pregnancy and so on. Setting the parameters of the interview at the outset avoids the situation where one professional misses the point and tries to do too much or too little.

When team members have been working together for some time, joint interviewing comes naturally. Initially, however, it is useful to agree who will lead the interview, and how the other professional will contribute (for example, should they wait for their comments to be invited or should they just chip in?). At the end of the interview, there should be an explicit agreement as to who is going to carry out each of the necessary tasks. We find it helpful to dictate a letter to the patient's general practitioner (GP) while the other professional is in the room (and often with the patient there as well), which allows discussion over the content. These letters set out the sequential thread of development of the treatment plan. Dictating the letter whilst sitting together means that the other professional can correct or elaborate on anything you write. It ensures that you share an understanding of the situation, that you both know what is meant to happen next and who is going to do it.

There are significant advantages to working in this way, but it does require alterations to the way that work is organised. In particular, this type of joint interviewing cannot be conducted in the setting of a traditional outpatient clinic. There are a number of other reasons to believe that traditional outpatient clinics have a limited utility, and this is explored in Chapter 9.

Consultation

We believe that psychiatrists work most effectively in teams when they follow the approach recommended in the UK Department of Health's Best Practice Guidance 'New Ways of Working for Psychiatrists' (Department of Health, 2005). This means that a significant part of their work involves consultation with other professionals rather than direct work with patients. This may involve one-to-one consultation, or providing a consultation function within multidisciplinary team meetings. Consultation can be more difficult than doing the work yourself, but it is worthwhile because it is efficient and it helps team members to develop their skills.

You can only offer consultation on problems if you have relevant expert knowledge and experience of dealing with similar situations. Neither knowledge nor experience is sufficient on its own. Knowledge that is entirely theoretical tends to guide you to advice that is difficult to implement or simply fails to work. Experience alone tends to guide you to advise others that they should do what you would do. However, in the absence of expert knowledge you rarely have enough information to know how you would deal with a situation, and in any case, what works for one practitioner does not necessarily work for everyone (because differences in personality determine different approaches to achieve the same ends). Furthermore, wisdom generated by experience decays quickly. As a general rule it is difficult to maintain good quality consultation skills unless you are also a practitioner.

Consultation is an interactive process. It rarely involves being directive or telling people exactly what to do. More often it involves determining the nature of the problem and an exploration of the range of potential solutions. It may involve a degree of direct advice and guidance, but it is essentially about facilitation. Potential solutions arise through dialogue, and they have to be refined through a kind of negotiation over what is ideal and what is possible. Consultation tends to work best when you have a continuing relationship with the other professional and a clear understanding of their concerns, their strengths, their weaknesses and the pressures upon them. In our experience one-off consultations with an unfamiliar expert are rarely helpful.

Where consultation works well, it involves a good deal of reflection, but it also comes to a conclusion. Both parties have to be clear as to what the conclusions are, and the action that needs to be taken. This means that there has to be sufficient time devoted to the task. The consultation has failed if the other person is left feeling criticised, or if they are unclear as to what they should be doing differently. An inconclusive consultation is not just unproductive, it can undermine rather than support the other professional.

The request for a consultation usually means that the other professional is anxious about something. An essential part of consultation is to reduce anxiety without dissipating responsibility. If a consultation makes the other professional less anxious because they have come to feel that everything will probably be all right, then there is a risk that all that has been shared is complacency. The outcome is more robust if their anxiety has reduced because they come to see the way forward more clearly.

Interfaces

Interfaces between teams cause problems. As patient care moves across team interfaces there is plenty of opportunity for everything to go wrong, and it often does. When there are problems within a team, they are likely to be evident in dysfunctional interactions with the rest of the world. Team interfaces have to be actively managed.

One of the sources of difficulty with interfaces is the natural tendency of any team to look inward and to become preoccupied with internal concerns and pressures. Teams easily feel embattled by the outside world, in which case they come to feel that *we* are doing a good job, but *they* are messing things up. Of course, this is sometimes true. The difficulty with them-versus-us feelings is that they lead you to build ever more robust defences against the outside world. This rarely solves any problems and in the long term tends to exacerbate them. It sometimes shifts problems from the team to someone else, but only temporarily.

Exclusion criteria are an example of a potentially destructive barricade against the outside world. In the UK, where CMHTs are publicly funded, they are expected to focus on helping people with severe and enduring mental health problems. They have finite resources to do this, which do not necessarily change as the number of patients increases and the pressure of work mounts. CMHTs have no alternative but to decline to offer a service to people who have mental health problems that are not severe and enduring. However, the definition of 'severe and enduring mental health problem' is inexact and it varies between locations and over time. This can create almost intolerable tensions between the CMHT and the GPs who refer to it. GPs refer patients who fall short of the criteria because they do not know what to do to help them. If the CMHT simply rejects referrals, writing back to the GP that the patient 'doesn't meet our criteria', the GP and the patient still have a problem. Some GPs will try to find another route into the CMHT for the patient, perhaps by making an inappropriate request for emergency assessment or by exaggerating patients' symptoms in referral letters. They certainly will come to feel alienated from the team, which has an impact when it is necessary for the CMHT to ask the GP to do something for them. Furthermore, in setting rigidly defensive boundaries around the team, it is inevitable that mistakes will be made, and that some people who need a service will be refused.

A more adaptive approach involves taking care to understand the referrer's perspective. When declining to offer a service, it is always a good idea to suggest an alternative solution, be this advice to the GP regarding treatment or suggesting a different agency that might be able to help (provided one is not simply suggesting an inappropriate referral to another team). Being prepared to discuss patients with referrers makes a huge difference. It improves their confidence in dealing with mental health problems and tends to reduce their referral rate. It can save time, effort and conflict if you agree to make an initial assessment of 'borderline cases' without making a commitment to provide a service, because it improves the credibility of the team and of the advice it gives. It also helps if the referrer can see that the team's defence of entry criteria is accompanied by a clear pay off, usually in terms of the ability to respond rapidly to emergencies. A similar use of engagement, discussion, flexibility and pay off are helpful at all the interfaces that the team has to manage.

Referral is only one aspect of the interface between CMHTs and primary care. When patients are under treatment by mental health teams, they remain in contact with GPs and other primary care professionals. Indeed, in the UK primary care retains some responsibility for the patient's mental health treatment even when a CMHT (including a psychiatrist) is involved. Consequently there is a need to actively manage the interface between CMHT and primary care during treatment. Most problems are a consequence of poor communication. If the GP is unaware of the treatment being given to the patient by the CMHT, or if he does not understand the rationale for it, then it is very difficult for him to make good decisions. There is little point in sending letters that exhaustively set out the content of mental health consultations. A succinct description of the plan and rationale is far more useful.

There are bound to be circumstances where patients turn up to see their GP with problems related to their mental illness or its treatment, for example because they are troubled by a drug side effect. Good communication is not just about providing up-to-date information. It is also about accessibility. As is the case with referrals, it makes a big difference if the psychiatrist or another relevant CMHT member is available to have a telephone discussion about problems. This works best where all team members either know, or can access, current plans for the entire case load. Although it is usually best to speak to the key worker, practicalities can make this difficult, and it is more important to give timely, well-informed advice than it is for the key worker to give the advice. This involves some effort for the CMHT but it is a worthwhile investment. Without access to advice, the GP has no choice but to make unilateral, uninformed decisions, which can be hugely disruptive to treatment.

There is little that can be done to prevent some types of interface problems, for example, the common and infuriating situation where general hospital specialists make inappropriate alterations to psychotropic medication. However, interface problems can be prevented most of the time with respect to primary care. The interface with primary care works a lot better when both parties can put faces to names. It is surprising how much difference occasional visits to GP surgeries can make. Making sure that treatment plans and their rationale are regularly communicated is important, but so too is clarity over the remit of the team and the way it works. GPs and other referrers who lack clarity over these matters can unwittingly create expectations with regard to treatment that are, in one way or another, unrealistic, and the result can be a confused and unhappy patient.

Boundary disputes

The next difficult interface issue is boundary disputes. These typically arise between CMHTs and other parts of the mental health service (such as child and adolescent services, forensic services, old age services, drug and alcohol services, learning disability services and so on) or between neighbouring CMHTs. The dispute is usually caused by clinical situations where the patient is close to a geographical or age boundary or has problems that straddle the remit of two teams. Occasionally a patient obviously needs help, but does not meet the criteria for any particular team. The unfortunate patient becomes a hot potato. Referrals unproductively pass between services and whoever is currently looking after them fails to develop a proper treatment plan because they feel that the patient is inappropriately placed. Sometimes no one will take responsibility and the patient does not get a service at all.

When managers are asked to prevent recurrent disputes of this sort, they usually set up meetings to clarify criteria for entry into the various teams. Although this is logical, it rarely resolves anything, and sometimes makes things worse (because criteria are defensively tightened, increasing the likelihood that patients will fail to meet any criteria). The only effective solution is goodwill, and an acceptance that all teams will have a small number of patients who for one reason or another do not perfectly fit within the team remit. A degree of reciprocal flexibility rarely leads to a movement of large numbers of patients from one service to another. However, reciprocity is hard to achieve, owing to the embattled, paranoid mood that prevails between many teams. We believe that excessive rigidity is essentially unprofessional and arguably unethical. Whilst a rigid position of non-negotiation may be satisfying in the context of a continuing struggle with another team, it is bound to act against the interests of the poor patient caught in the middle.

Transfers of care

Transfers of care between teams are inevitable, because people change addresses, and because patients have different needs at different times. Transfers are a key moment when interventions go wrong. They have to be timely, so that the overall coherence of treatment is maintained. Organisational pressures can encourage hurried or long delayed transfers, but there is a responsibility on both teams to try to avoid this, because they both cause serious problems for the patient. Adequate information needs to travel ahead of the patient, both in terms of history and what has gone before, and more importantly the overall treatment strategy. Patients need time to understand why a transfer is desirable, but also sufficient time to end their relationship with the current team, so that they do not experience a confusing discontinuity of treatment.

This advice is a counsel of perfection and as such it may be hard to follow. Indeed, unsatisfactory transfers of care seem to be more frequent than they used to be. This is probably a consequence of the proliferation of specialist teams, increasingly pro-grammatic treatment regimes, and the new mixed economy of mental health care. This does not mean that the effects cannot be ameliorated. For example, health insurance coverage will sometimes be exhausted during private treatment, and the National Health Service (NHS) then has to take over. However, this is a foreseeable event and there is no reason why the transfer should occur at very short notice and without planning. Indeed prior warning to the receiving team of a transfer of care usually prevents problems.

Liaising with external agencies

It can be very difficult to work at the interface with external agencies, especially those that lack expertise in mental health problems. They often have very different values or a different agenda from your own. Mental health professionals in the UK have to participate in child protection meetings and in Multi-Agency Public Protection Arrangements (MAPPAs) concerning their patients. These are large meetings that involve health professionals, police, social services and probation. Getting all the agencies together to talk where there is concern that a person could be dangerous to a child or to the public seems like a self-evidently good idea. In fact there have been cogent criticisms of both processes, and their effectiveness in preventing harm is open to question. However, they are unlikely to be abolished and we are obliged to attend them.

Quite apart from the question of whether large meetings of professionals are the best way to protect third parties, these meetings work to an uncertain set of rules and values. Each agency has a different approach with regard to confidentiality. They have different priorities and have a varying concern for the welfare of the index person. Representatives from different agencies do not necessarily understand the information that is shared. A child protection social worker or a police officer may have little knowledge about mental health and may easily misunderstand the terms we use. In ordinary vocabulary, 'psychotic' implies wildly deranged and dangerous and 'borderline personality disorder' seems to indicate a mild problem which is almost within normal limits.

When participating in these meetings, teams have to be true to their own professional and ethical obligations, which can be surprisingly difficult when the general level of anxiety about the person starts to rise. These meetings should be attended by senior professionals, usually in pairs. There is no value in being needlessly obstructive, but some care is needed in making a contribution, so that confidences are not unnecessarily broken, and to ensure that everyone understands what has been said. At the end of the meeting it is wise to be absolutely explicit as to what actions your own team is going to take, as it is common to find that the chair has misunderstood. It is particularly important to approve and, if necessary, correct the minutes. These become legal records and as such they can become vehicles for propagating inaccuracies and misconceptions.

'Discharge to consultant'

The final interface issue of note concerns the discharge of patients. When people suffering from mental health problems get better, they should be discharged unless there is a good reason not to. This is explored more fully in Chapter 16. The issue of relevance to teamwork is the practice known as 'discharge to consultant'. This happens when the patient has made sufficient progress under the team such that active treatment is completed. Rather than discharge the patient from the team completely, they are given appointments to see the psychiatrist. This is intrinsically dysfunctional, unless there is a specific task for the psychiatrist to carry out. It gives an ambiguous message to the patient with regard to the team's confidence that their improved mental health will endure, and it holds them in the status of psychiatric patient. It moves the psychiatrist away from focussed work, back towards fruitless routine clinics. It invites the psychiatrist to react unnecessarily to changes in the patient's frame of mind. There is not a jot of evidence that infrequent outpatient appointments provide meaningful monitoring that might prevent relapse. Indeed, in our experience, full discharge and an easy route back into the service is much more effective in this regard. Timely responses to requests for help are more possible if the psychiatrist is not tied up with clinics full of patients who are essentially well. 'Discharge to consultant' is a route back to an older, less effective style of teamwork.

Team building

Effective teams have a set of shared values and clinical concepts that facilitate functional relationships between team members. These constitute the team culture. A positive team culture is more likely to develop where there is attention to team building. There are many ways of building a team culture, but we believe that there are a few simple measures that make it much easier.
* The key senior professionals in the team, which may be just two people, need to foster their relationship. This means spending time talking things through on a regular basis. At the very least this allows points of disagreement to be resolved without dragging the whole team into a difficult process of warring leaders. In any case,

dialogue works better than group discussion in crystallising thinking, and if the leaders have a clear set of ideas in common, this is bound to spread to the rest of the team.

- Teams benefit from having some 'downtime' together, periods at lunch or at the end of the day when they have time to talk over the day's activity, or just to be together for a cup of coffee. Not everyone likes this, but these informal times make an important contribution to team relationships. Doctors often hold themselves aloof from these activities, which is usually a mistake. Downtime creates an environment where team culture can develop.

- Joint working, for example, multidisciplinary assessment, spreads team culture if everyone works with everyone else from time to time.

- Change keeps teams alive, provided it is initiated from within the team (there is nothing intrinsically wrong with externally driven change, but it makes little contribution to team building). If a team comes to believe that change is unnecessary, that it has achieved an end point of excellence, then the service becomes resistant to improvement. However, no team functions so well that it cannot be improved. People may like working in comfortably unchanging environments, but this type of comfort is stagnation.

The standard managerial approach to team building is to organise 'away-days'. There is a certain irony in the use of this term, as British Rail used to market tickets for return journeys as 'Awaydays', inviting the observation that with away-days you travel but you end up where you started. Taking the whole team away from work for a day to talk about itself is a costly business. The exercise can be worthwhile if the day involves the whole team understanding and owning problems, in order to get everyone to contribute to plans. There is only a point to this if the team has the authority to implement the plans it comes up with. There is always a risk that these days will provide a focus for cynicism and lead to an acting out of team tensions. This is much less likely to happen if there are specific tasks set beforehand. Away-days should be facilitated by a well-briefed outsider, who should be aware of any individual who is likely to try to use the occasion as a platform for grievances. It is usually necessary to involve all team members in specific tasks in the course of the day, and to prevent formal leaders from dominating the proceedings.

Responsibility

Responsibility is a potentially corrosive issue in teams. The responsibilities of a psychiatrist working alone are clear and are set out in the codes of bodies such as the General Medical Council (GMC). In teams it is all much more ambiguous.

One of the obstructions in developing CMHT working in the UK has been the belief amongst some doctors that they hold clinical and ethical responsibility for the work of the whole team. They have been reluctant to hand over the task of assessment and decision making to other professions, in the belief that they remain responsible even if they have had no direct contact with the patient. Although this is not correct, there are ambiguous areas. On the one hand, qualified professionals are individually responsible (and liable) for their own actions. This includes ensuring that they do not work outside of their area of competence. On the other hand, doctors do have responsibility for the advice they give to other team members. They have special legal responsibilities for patients when they are inpatients, irrespective of whether they are legally detained. The existence of ambiguities over responsibility means that the issue can become a battleground when there are problems in a team.

Sometimes psychiatrists have to insist on their point of view, because they sincerely believe that something bad will happen if they are ignored. This does not excuse those psychiatrists who insist that they should always prevail because they are 'ultimately responsible'. Teams cannot function if one person tries to dominate and control everything. Consequently, when other professionals find themselves working with controlling psychiatrists, they almost invariably cope with the situation through secrecy and subversion. They avoid inappropriate control by manipulating the psychiatrist. They are careful what they tell him, and avoid joint working. The pattern is dysfunctional and inherently dangerous.

We have put some emphasis on the ways in which psychiatrists can disrupt teams, but other disciplines are equally capable of causing problems. Nurses can have particular difficulty in working autonomously and accepting responsibility. This becomes evident in a common dysfunctional behaviour known to us as 'the nurse cop-out'. This is based on the belief that once a doctor is aware of a problem, the nurse bears no further responsibility. What happens is that the nurse wants to discuss every patient on their case load very regularly, whether or not there is a decision to be made. This allows them to write 'Discussed with Dr X' in their notes, which in their mind absolves them of responsibility if anything goes wrong. There are variations on this theme such as insisting that you see the patient in order to make a decision that could be made equally well through a discussion between professionals.

At one level, this pattern of behaviour is irritating and wastes time. However, it reflects a deeper problem, and as such it demands action. The process of absolving oneself of responsibility is an invitation to ill-considered (and irresponsible) decision making. Accountability for one's actions is an essential stimulus to serious and careful thinking. The cop-out is not a behaviour that can be tolerated within a team.

Group dynamics

The biggest pitfall relating to responsibility in teams is the effect of group dynamics. These are emergent characteristics of whole teams, and they can cause real problems despite the fact that each individual member of the team acts appropriately. We are all prey to group processes and their effects can go unnoticed if you are not attentive to them.

When risk issues are discussed as a group, it is easy for objectivity to be lost. Take the example of a well-known patient who unexpectedly says that he has been thinking of suicide, and that if he killed himself he would have to kill his children too. Obviously, the prospect of a homicide-suicide is dreadful, and whilst such events are rare, they do happen. It is hard to accept that someone you know and like might act in this way. Taking action makes it clear to the patient that you think he is potentially dangerous to his children. Once someone in the team expresses a view that 'he wouldn't do something like that', there is a strong temptation for other team members to express similar views, and for the whole team to be moved to complacency, because it is comforting. However, 'he wouldn't do something like that' is not a valid contribution to the assessment of risk. The real question is 'What restraining factors exist and are they sufficient to delay action?' In this example, one should take the risk very seriously, and there are very few reasons not to take firm action. Once group complacency has taken hold, it can be difficult to retain this perspective.

Similar but converse processes can lead to team panic over risk, whereby an objectively small risk, often concerning an unpopular patient, leads to rising team anxiety. The outcome is usually an inappropriate referral of the patient out of the team, for example, to a forensic psychiatry service. This does little to help the patient or to reduce risk, as the other service is likely to resist the referral and in the process treatment plans go into a state of suspension. The only protection against team complacency and team panic is to look out for them, which is a responsibility of each team member.

Awestruck teams

Another problematic group dynamic is the awestruck team. This can look benign but is actually dysfunctional. It arises where one team member is generally regarded as much more competent than everybody else, and the team increasingly looks to him to generate treatment plans. Whilst the dominant person may be a psychiatrist, it can be someone from any profession. Teams do not become awestruck through bullying or deliberate domination. Indeed, awestruck teams are often happy to be so, because the dominant person is likely to be objectively able, charismatic and of high status. Such individuals invariably talk a good talk. However, if they are generating all the ideas and whole treatment plans, they are actually causing a major problem. There is no level of outstanding ability that allows any professional to have all the good ideas all of the time. It is inevitable that this dominant professional will generate ideas and plans that are less than ideal for at least some patients. Behind apparently sophisticated expositions, the dominant person is likely to be relying upon a narrow range of inflexible schemata. The dynamic makes the team increasingly dependent and unable to function in the absence of the dominant person.

Awestruckness is best tackled by the dominant person, who has to learn to keep his mouth shut some of the time. He has to resist forever leaping ahead of everyone else in discussions, because less able team members will generate good ideas if they are given time to do so. Unfortunately it can be very difficult to recognise that you are dominating a team in this way, so other team members have to be prepared to point out what is happening.

Main points in this chapter

1. Joint working in teams works much better than parallel working.
2. Interfaces with other teams work best where you understand other teams' perspectives, try to help them to solve problems, remain accessible to them and keep them well informed.
3. Team building occurs more effectively in small activities that happen every day than in set-piece isolated events.
4. 'Good' teams can develop dysfunctional group dynamics. These can be controlled if you are attentive to them.

7 Inpatient treatment in the era of community psychiatry

Twenty years of rapid and continuing change in mental health services have brought us to the point where, in the UK and in many other countries, we are unequivocally in the era of community psychiatry. The provision of treatment in, or close to, the patient's home is the dominant model of practice, with empirical evidence to support its advantages and a balance of opinion that suggests it is preferred by service users (e.g. Dean *et al.*, 1993; Burns *et al.*, 2001). However, inpatient care shows no sign of disappearing. The historical trend in the UK for national bed numbers to drop has reversed. This has gone largely unnoticed, as the new beds (which now represent over fifty percent of the total) are in a new state-funded private sector (Ryan *et al.*, 2007). For various reasons, including high cost, inpatient treatment continues to attract concern, but little attention has been paid to admission as a necessary part of some people's treatment.

Generally speaking, most psychiatrists are discernibly either enthusiasts or skeptics with regard to new models of care. This climate of opinion tends to obscure the question of the location of care as an important component to every strategic treatment plan. It is hard to find an appropriate role for inpatient stays as part of a coherent treatment strategy if one is preoccupied with either keeping patients out of hospital at all costs or trying to overcome barriers to admission. Inpatient treatment is unlikely to be a constructive component of care if it is either the option of last resort or the centrepiece of longer term treatment.

If one considers the possible advantages of inpatient treatment over other modalities of care, there are three significant factors that are rhetorically defensible. The first is that inpatient care gives mental health professionals control over the patient. The second is that twenty-four hour observation may improve assessment. The third is that twenty-four hour treatment may be more intense than other forms of treatment. All of these factors can have a legitimate role in treatment, but they each have major limitations.

Control

The question of control represents a dilemma at the heart of psychiatric practice. People who are mentally ill lose control of their lives, and helping them to regain this is a key objective of treatment. However, suicidal ideas, aggression, loss of judgement and lack of insight are features of some of the disorders that we treat. This means that we try to control our patients to a greater or lesser extent in the course of a proportion of treatments. If we did not do this, many patients would come to serious harm before they had a chance to recover (sometimes through causing harm to others), and some patients would receive no treatment at all. However, individual freedom is a high order value in a democracy. Baldly stating that mental health professionals routinely seek to control patients is an affront to the liberal and libertarian sensibilities that many of us hold dear. In addition to this, good mental health means managing your own well being. A loss of symptoms that is contingent on a loss of freedom can only be regarded as partial recovery at best. If treatment is to improve patients' lives, we have to move from control to personal autonomy as treatment progresses.

Control by staff is a prominent feature of inpatient units. Patients who accept treatment of their own volition are equally subject to staff control as those who are legally detained, the difference between them being the degree of duress to which they are subjected. The key element of control in this setting is the loss of freedom of movement. Patients have to ask permission to leave inpatient units, which inevitably means that a whole range of other freedoms are lost. They have little choice but to submit to institutional routines of mealtimes, medication rounds, bedtimes and rising times. No matter how benign such a regime may be, it traps patients in an unfamiliar routine with few choices available to them. It is hardly surprising that many people find this oppressive. Such a loss of autonomy is intrinsically counter-productive to the task of helping them to manage their lives and their illnesses.

Of course, some patients value the certainties of an institutional existence. It can be a relief to seek asylum from life's stresses. This was, after all, the rationale for lunatic asylums when they were first established in the nineteenth century. There is still a widespread belief that asylum is one of the therapeutic advantages of inpatient treatment. However, few difficulties in life improve when they are neglected, and there is a steep and slippery slope into avoidance and dependency. Living under such a regime for months or years is bound to lead to institutionalisation, which is damaging to people who are mentally well (as may happen to long-term prisoners), and is known to exacerbate the effects of chronic mental illness.

Set against all of this is the fact that during inpatient stays the consequences of hopelessness, disinhibition, aggression and self-neglect can be contained. Having taken control of the administration of medication, it is possible to ensure that it is taken and to be certain of its effects. In terms of both short-term decision making and long-term treatment strategies, the key questions are 'How much control do we need? For how long? What are the predictable adverse consequences of this degree of control? How can they be ameliorated? Is there a safe and credible alternative?' The answers to these questions can be counter-intuitive, as they do not necessarily depend on the severity of the illness. Many people with florid schizophreniform psychosis are not greatly at risk, and can be safely treated in their own homes with intensive community support. On the other hand even relatively mild degrees of mania impair people's judgement through over-expansiveness and disinhibition. If people with hypomania are left to their own devices for any length of time, they can make devastatingly bad judgements, for example, with regard to their financial situation or their sexual behaviour.

Assessment

In the past patients were commonly admitted solely for the purpose of assessment. There is no doubt that one can make a better assessment of a patient's mental state in the hospital setting compared with an outpatient interview. However, under most circumstances neither is as effective as assessing the patient at home. Admission to hospital for assessment is a bit like pinning a butterfly to a piece of card. It may allow you to get a really good look, but everything is taken out of context. If mental illness happens in peoples' lives as much as in their minds, then assessing them in their own environment must be the location of choice. In addition to this, admission to hospital induces changes in people's behaviour, so that assessment as an inpatient can be misleading.

There are some exceptions to this general rule. If a patient is very isolated and suffering from a disorder (such as cognitive impairment or severe thought disorder) that makes history taking very difficult, then there may be little alternative to assessment in hospital (though this must be set against the risk that the patient might become more confused and muddled in a strange environment). Assessment is sometimes best carried out in hospital because the present environment is highly unsatisfactory, as may be the case when prisoners show signs of serious mental illness. Patients whose illness leads them to wander can be impossible to assess without admission. When someone is engaging in recurrent antisocial behaviour, there can be real ambiguity as to whether they are suffering from psychosis, personality disorder or both, and admission may be the most effective way of confirming or excluding the presence of serious illness.

Notwithstanding these exceptions, admission to hospital for assessment should be undertaken with caution. It is unlikely to resolve anything unless you are clear as to what you are expecting to see in order to test your initial hypothesis, and are quite certain that the necessary assessment is within the capabilities of the inpatient staff.

Intensive treatment

It should be possible (if only in theory) to organise especially intensive forms of treatment in inpatient settings. Certainly there are historical examples of this. Twenty-five years ago the therapeutic community movement was highly influential in British inpatient care. The concept was pioneered by Maxwell Jones and others at the Henderson Hospital and in other parts of the NHS. These projects had a significant influence on later developments in community psychiatry. The idea of therapeutic communities was that change could arise from the experience of living and working together in a 'democratic' structure, with daily groups to reflect on the experience. Working in a therapeutic community was an interesting and intense experience. However, changes in priorities and funding arrangements have almost eliminated therapeutic communities from NHS practice (although they are alive and well in other settings designed to encourage change). There is some evidence that therapeutic communities may be effective in altering the behaviour of people with severe personality problems, though a recent attempt to replicate the Henderson Hospital regime in other parts of the UK has not been an unqualified success.

Similarly, there are a handful of inpatient units that specialise in intensive behavioural treatments. Some of these offer specialist inpatient behaviour therapy for conditions such as severe obsessive-compulsive disorder. Others offer behaviour modification regimes for people with brain injuries or learning disabilities. There are a number of private units specialising in behavioural/psychotherapeutic treatment of eating disorders. There is little doubt that these intensive therapies induce change in people. What is more difficult is the question as to whether those changes persist and generalise when the patient moves out of a highly structured environment.

The final model of intensive inpatient treatment is the social rehabilitation regimes that were developed in institutions such as Netherne Hospital in Surrey (this was the hospital described in Wing and Brown's 1970 seminal work on the impact of the inpatient environment on patients suffering from chronic schizophrenia, the so-called 'Three Hospitals' study). These offered a long-term, staged approach to rehabilitation, mainly aimed at overcoming the combined effects of chronic psychosis and institutionalisation. Inpatient rehabilitation has all but disappeared from the NHS. The new private sector offers inpatient care for these patients, but there is serious doubt as to the nature of its rehabilitation regimes, or, in many cases, whether it offers rehabilitation at all (Poole *et al.*, 2002).

There is variation in the strength of the evidence supporting these intensive inpatient treatments. What is really striking is that nearly all forms of intensive inpatient treatment have disappeared from the NHS, partly due to a loss of faith in inpatient treatment in general. Similar, if slower, changes have occurred in countries where mental health care is mainly paid for by insurers. It would appear that intensive treatment is not commonly available in modern inpatient units. Indeed, there is a great deal of concern at present over a perception that NHS inpatient units lack therapeutic activity, or that they may be positively anti-therapeutic.

Inpatient units as therapeutic environments

The discussion so far brings us to the point where it appears that the only real advantages of modern inpatient care concern control and containment. To make things worse, there is a general perception that modern acute inpatient units are less pleasant environments than the corresponding wards in old-fashioned mental hospitals. The exploration of this deterioration in inpatient environments does, we think, give some clues about the nature of inpatient admissions as therapeutic interventions.

County asylums were grand municipal buildings with a sort of austere beauty, located in spacious grounds. The majority of the residents lived in back wards, barren long-stay units that offered little prospect of improvement or discharge. The acute short-stay wards, on the other hand, tended to be more comfortable. They were a focus of a lot of activity, and patients had a degree of privacy. There usually were good facilities for exercise and a host of diversional activities. There was rarely any great pressure on beds, admissions proceeded in a leisurely fashion and they offered a retreat from the stresses and strains of life. It must be said that they were generally located far from patients' homes, and visiting could be difficult. There was also an 'under-life', as there is in all institutions. Women often faced sexual harassment or worse from males and there were commonly problems of bullying (whether by other patients or by abusive staff). Decisions regarding discharge were very dependent on alterations in mental state rather than more functional assessments, because mental state was all that could be assessed in these decontextualised settings.

Modern inpatient units, on the other hand, are rarely well designed. They tend to be cheaply constructed, and crammed into a corner of a general hospital site, with little open space and with inadequate internal space to allow for privacy, peace and quiet, or diversional activity. There is constant pressure on beds, so that they tend to be continuously full or over-occupied, with patients on leave sharing beds with the newly admitted. A high proportion of patients are legally detained and many are severely unwell. Combined with an overall lack of space, this can create a 'pressure cooker' atmosphere, and many patients feel intimidated by other disturbed people. There are problems with patients returning to the ward intoxicated with alcohol, and cannabis (and occasionally other drugs) circulates amongst younger patients. Patients complain of boredom and inactivity, and the liveliest place in the unit is likely to be the smoking area.

Nearly all of the most interesting service developments of recent years have occurred in community teams, and there has been a massive expansion in the number of jobs for mental health professionals in the community. This has drawn staff away from inpatient areas. The paradox is that successful community treatment depends on the inpatient area being well integrated with community teams, in order to allow overarching treatment strategies to be pursued through inpatient stays and beyond. There are still many high quality inpatient nurses. There is also a disproportionate number of recently qualified staff on wards who intend to move on, and a rump of staff with significant limitations, who remain as inpatient nurses because this allows close supervision of their work. Together with the intrinsic problems of shift working, this staff mix can create real difficulties in achieving consistency in treatment plans or even accurate information about what has been happening to a patient. There are few more frustrating experiences than arranging to review a patient's treatment, only to be told 'Sorry, I can't tell you much about him because I've been off for four days'. Treatment plans can be derailed by the small deviations that some staff employ to have a quiet life, for example, the overuse of night sedation and 'confusion' over legal powers (e.g. 'Sorry, he hasn't had any medication but we can't force him to have treatment under section 2 of the Mental Health Act').

Some of the problems of modern inpatient care set out above were equally true of inpatient care in asylums. There is a general belief amongst hospital managers in the UK that the problem of poor inpatient environments can be resolved by planning for discharge from the day of admission, and by providing specific therapies to inpatients, essentially meaning psychological therapies. We do not believe that either is necessarily possible or desirable. Discharge plans can be difficult to make until the effects of treatment are evident. Few psychological therapies are effective if they are commenced during the most severe phase of illness, and some are contraindicated at that point. We believe that two factors can improve inpatient care. One is the location and physical structure of the building, which should be close to the patient's home and with sufficient space to create a decent living and treatment environment. The other is close integration of community and inpatient staff, who should function as a single team.

It appears to us that what has been lost in recent thinking has been an awareness of the importance of bread and butter nursing, skilled but not programmatic. The present low regard for its importance is clearly indicated by the increasing proportion of inpatient nursing care that is delivered by untrained nursing assistants (some of whom are highly skilled, but some of whom most certainly are not). Equally, the trend towards treatment pathways and programmes of care has somewhat obscured the power of non-specific aspects of treatment, which includes activities for inpatients, such as exercise, that are generally a good thing but do not have a specific therapeutic aim.

The superiority of community over institutional psychiatry seems to us to be overwhelming. This belief is not based on the scientific evidence (which is equivocal) but arises from the personal experience of working in both systems (which has been absolutely unambiguous). We are concerned by the present trend that seems to be pushing us back towards more custodial forms of care. We strongly believe that hospital admissions should be avoided if possible and that, generally speaking, lengthy admissions are counter-productive. Nonetheless, it seems to us that there *is* a specific therapeutic value to inpatient stays for some patients at some times, and that this is enhanced if due attention is paid to avoiding factors that tend towards an anti-therapeutic atmosphere, which includes conspicuous and intimidating security measures.

Inpatient stays require active management, so that one anticipates next steps in the face of developments. Pressing to get patients out of hospital as soon as they show a glimmer of improvement is rarely the best strategy, unless this forms part of a thought-through plan with the community team. Occasionally, longer stays are appropriate and productive. Some very disabled patients, such as people who have slipped into vagrancy because of long untreated psychosis, show a surprising range of improvements (both symptomatic and functional) after three months or more in hospital, even where the initial improvement in symptoms has occurred quite promptly.

The course of inpatient episodes

One aspect of inpatient care that has been neglected in the general pressure to minimise the length of admissions has been serious and rational thinking about the course and structure of inpatient episodes. There is a big difference between thoughtful planning to avoid unproductively long admissions and the common practice of daily urgency to discharge. The problem with the latter approach is that it is only effective in overcoming the tendency of some weak clinicians to preside over lengthy and directionless admissions. Most of the time, it has little effect on length of stay, and may in fact lengthen it by interfering with more considered planning.

As a rule of thumb, an admission that lasts a few days is pointless. If sufficient progress can be made to allow an appropriate discharge in a week, then it is highly unlikely that the patient was so severely ill or at risk as to justify the admission in the first instance. All of the adverse effects of admission, including damage to the therapeutic relationship with the team, tend to arise early in inpatient stays. This means that short admissions tend to dictate a preponderance of negative effects over positive therapeutic gains. In our experience, the majority of fruitful admissions last between three to six weeks in total. There is an initial crisis phase, when the patient is very ill, and sometimes legally detained, during which it is important to be clear with the patient about what you are doing and why. A substantial proportion of patients feel that they have been incarcerated when they are admitted to hospital, and indefinite incarceration is frightening. Whilst it is usually a mistake to be very specific about the likely discharge date (because events can alter plans, and there is nothing so damaging to a therapeutic relationship as the perception that you have lied), some clarity over the likely course of the admission makes the experience less oppressive, and naturally enough people are then less likely to rail against the injustice of their predicament. Such railing is entirely understandable, but it is an obstruction to the task of getting the patient better whilst trying to ameliorate or undo the damage done to the relationship with the team.

The practice of sending patients home for gradually increasing periods of leave during the second half of the admission is very common, and it is a prominent feature of our own practice. One could argue that, if the main advantage of admission is control and containment, then sending the patient home for substantial periods is nonsense. However, there are major problems with the transition between inpatient and community treatment. It is well established that a key risk time for suicide is the first month after discharge. Furthermore, there is a real challenge around the task of ensuring that symptomatic improvements persist after discharge. The new Crisis Resolution and Home Treatment teams have a remit to facilitate early discharge, but it has yet to be seen whether their capacity to offer intensive input will outweigh the disruption of repeated changes of personnel over short periods of time.

It is too simple minded to suppose that issues of control evaporate when the patient goes home for a while. The advantage of incremental leave is that it greatly enhances continuity between inpatient and community care. Where patients already have a community key worker ('care co-ordinator' in the current UK jargon), then it is best if they are closely involved in the management of the admission. This includes involvement in making plans, seeing the patient regularly in hospital and visiting during periods of leave. Where the patient is introduced to community staff for the first time, a similar involvement of a new key worker at an early stage makes discharge planning far easier.

Integration of inpatient and community treatment

It is believed by many community psychiatrists, including ourselves, that integration and continuity of care are major advantages of British mental health services (Burns & Priebe, 1999). However, perhaps following the dominant international model, some services are developing separate community and inpatient mental health teams, with dedicated consultant psychiatrists whose job is exclusively concerned with inpatient treatment. These developments have some vocal advocates. The advantages are said to be that:

- nursing staff are not tied up with multiple ward reviews in the course of the week,
- discharges can occur more promptly because there is no delay waiting for the consultant psychiatrist's weekly visit, and
- the leadership of a consultant psychiatrist has a positive impact on the therapeutic quality of the ward.

We believe that these advantages are illusory, as they are based on a poor model of inpatient care (is it seriously suggested, for example, that the patient should be discharged the day the auditory hallucinations stop and that a consultant psychiatrist should be on hand to detect this?), which is patronising in its attitude to nurses and other non-medical professionals, needlessly casts aside the considerable strengths of a more integrated approach and offers a pattern of working for the inpatient consultant that is unsustainable over years.

However, there is a real issue about ward reviews or 'ward rounds'. The subject is worth exploring because, when patients are asked, they consistently rank the weekly ward round amongst the most unpleasant and stressful aspects of inpatient treatment. Furthermore, the discussion illuminates some issues concerning the ways that teams can organise themselves to optimise constructive admissions.

Traditional British ward rounds are based on an implicit model that puts the consultant psychiatrist at the centre of decision making. This has its origins in the deeply ingrained hierarchal structure of health care, but is strongly supported by common law and statutory responsibilities whereby the consultant has a specific bottom-line responsibility for inpatient care. In their grandest form, ward rounds are lengthy meetings that are attended by everyone who has a contribution to make to the consultant's task of assessment and decision making. Junior doctors and nursing staff are invariably present. There may be occupational therapists, social workers and community key workers in attendance. As ward rounds are the main clinical meeting of the week, they are often a focus for teaching. Students from any, or all, of the relevant disciplines may wish to attend. A minimal ward round might have four mental health professionals in attendance. It is not uncommon to have ten professionals in the room at any one time.

Patients are discussed in turn. There may not be an agenda, so that patients wait apprehensively, uncertain as to when they will be seen. Partners, relatives and friends often attend, and are usually kept waiting for long periods. After the initial discussion, the unfortunate patient comes in to be interviewed. In theory, this gives them an opportunity to discuss and negotiate treatment plans, but the setting is intrinsically daunting and many people feel intimidated. Talking about difficult feelings and experiences in front of a large group of people is humiliating. The development of patient advocacy services has helped patients to articulate their wishes to these meetings, but this too adds to the number of people in attendance. No matter how much effort is made to be user friendly, ward rounds are bound to be difficult for patients.

We have been unhappy with ward rounds ever since we became consultants, but our personal efforts to reform the process only ever ameliorated their worst aspects.

Box 7.1 Legitimate functions of 'ward rounds'

- To allow regular contact between consultant psychiatrist and patients
- To allow patient involvement in treatment planning
- To allow regular contact between community key worker and inpatient
- To allow the community key worker to be involved in, or preferably to lead, inpatient treatment planning (in the belief that this improves the integration of inpatient and community treatment plans)
- To allow inpatient staff to be involved in treatment planning and to be able to recognise how their interventions fit into a long-term strategy
- To provide a real-life focus for teaching

Generally speaking, changes to ward rounds led by psychiatrists tend to drift back to the status quo ante. In retrospect, these efforts were naive, because the central flaw of ward rounds is precisely their focus on the needs of the consultant, not the needs of the patient or the team. The consultant is thus in a very weak position to lead fundamental change. The key to improving practice has been to give the task of finding a solution to the patients and the team. In our opinion, it is this process that is important rather than any specific solution.

One of us has been through such a process twice in recent years, in two locations with very different service configurations. In each case, changes were devised primarily by the CMHT and ward managers. Patient opinion was similar on both occasions. On the whole, they wanted regular contact with the consultant psychiatrist, who was seen as being in charge. They did want choices and involvement in decisions about their treatment. They definitely did not want to be 'paraded' in front of massed professionals, though they were fairly relaxed about the presence of staff who they knew and who had direct and continuing involvement with them.

Box 7.1 sets out the legitimate functions of ward rounds that must be attended to if they are to be reformed. The solutions that we have seen work have been dictated by the specific circumstances of the services concerned. They are described here to illustrate this, not as recommendations of 'best practice'.

The first service was located in a free-standing building within the area it served. As the CMHT office and the inpatient beds were in the same place, it was easy for the community staff to remain in contact with their patients during inpatient stays. The community team leader and the ward manager met once a week, a day before the ward round. The two managers consulted with their staff and jointly made long- and short-term plans for patients' care. They drew up a timetabled agenda for the ward round, with specific tasks for the consultant to carry out. If a plan was proceeding satisfactorily, and there were no decisions to be made, patients were asked if they wished to see the consultant. They could be seen alone or with an advocate if they wanted. Patients on leave were reviewed at home, not in hospital. Ward rounds became briefer and more focussed. There was a discernible improvement in the quality of plans. Patients seemed to feel less exposed by the process.

The second service had a CMHT base in the area it served, but the inpatient unit was thirteen miles away. Community key workers visited their patients in hospital early in the week in order to assess their progress and to discuss further plans with them. They then led discussion at a midweek meeting at the CMHT base, which was also attended by a member of the inpatient staff. If patients were on leave, they were reviewed at home after the meeting. Out of the discussion, plans were made, and the consultant was given specific tasks to carry out when he saw the patient with the inpatient nurse the next day. His task could be to make a treatment plan on the basis of the interview where, for example, his skills were needed to resolve diagnostic uncertainty. In the absence of a specific task, patients were given the choice as to whether to see the consultant.

In both cases, the arrangements were seen to be successful, and overall were neutral in terms of demand on staff time. In both cases, teaching suffered, and alternative arrangements had to be made for students. There was some tendency to drift back towards the old pattern, which was familiar and comfortable. All service developments are vulnerable to this, and any change in working practice has to be supported by giving someone specific responsibility to be vigilant against a quiet return to old habits.

Inappropriate and overextended admissions

Many problems in clinical practice have their origins very early in treatment or are due to the rigidity of organisational systems. Inappropriate and overlong admissions almost invariably are due to one or other of these. However, it is impossible to completely eliminate admissions that are unnecessary or overextended and a system achieving this would probably also prevent some appropriate admissions.

A significant proportion of patients are admitted out of hours and without the involvement of the local team. Despite attempts to improve out-of-hours assessment and crisis response, the task still tends to fall to hospital-based medical staff, who are inexperienced. Such staff have an understandable tendency to admit people 'just in case'. Unable to guarantee a timely and appropriate intervention from another part of the service, they err on the side of caution and admit. Such admissions can appear highly inappropriate to more senior professionals reviewing the patient the next day, because they have a greater awareness of (and faith in) alternative interventions.

It is easier to avoid admitting someone in the first place than it is to discharge them quickly once they have been admitted. Once a person is in hospital, the service's responsibilities towards them change substantially. There is little alternative but to carry out a full assessment of someone who has been admitted, and this takes days in most cases. Duty doctors often write rather defensively in the notes to the effect 'admitted overnight for assessment', but this is a fantasy. Once the person is in hospital, institutional imperatives take over.

The fault here lies in systems. If you put inexperienced professionals in isolated positions and ask them to make decisions, they are always likely to be overcautious. It would be better to take inexperienced professionals out of the situation, and ensure that every patient is assessed by an experienced clinician. This is a difficult aspiration to realise in the face of the expense of maintaining twenty-four hour staffing of an emergency system (especially as staff are inactive for most the night shift; a surprisingly small number of people present in need of urgent assessment at night). However, Crisis Resolution and Home Treatment teams attempt to achieve this, but they only achieve modest reductions in admissions (Glover *et al.*, 2006). It is only realistic, we would suggest, to expect 'inappropriate admissions' and deal with them efficiently. Putting great energy into avoiding them completely is probably futile.

A small proportion of 'inappropriate admissions' occur because people who are not mentally ill want to hide out in hospital. These are individuals with other types of problems who try to use psychiatric admission as an inappropriate coping strategy. This includes people facing criminal charges, people who become homeless, and people who face financial crisis. The awareness of this creates a degree of vigilance amongst staff for stories that are uncorroborated or inconsistent, symptoms that seem inauthentic, and evasive responses to questions. Amongst the group of patients whose behaviour raises such suspicions, there is a group of mentally ill people with an atypical or complicated presentation.

These situations tend to polarise opinion amongst staff between those who are outraged at apparent attempts at deception and those who are more cautious in coming to conclusions (often the psychiatrists because, at the end of the day, it is they who are most likely to take the rap if a misjudgement is made and things go wrong). Such splits are an impediment to sensible practice. One group tends to be drawn towards angry confrontation, whilst the other acts as if the patient is ill until proven otherwise. Different members of staff adopt different stances, which is wildly dysfunctional. What works far better is openness and honesty with the patient, which is compatible with both opinions, and is in any case a first principle of therapeutic relationships. The staff group has to agree on a position whereby members share the ambiguities with the patient and explain how they intend to resolve them. This is a far better option than a protracted struggle between staff members which helps no one, least of all the patient.

Over-extended inpatient episodes can occur because patients do not respond to standard treatments or they develop a physical illness or there is some other complication to the clinical situation. There is little that anyone can do to avoid this happening from time to time. However, many other overextended admissions occur because there has been a lack of clarity over treatment plans at the beginning. For example, admitting a patient because you do not know what to do next is a strategy that is bound to fail. Bereft of a clear plan at the outset, inpatient treatment is unlikely to resolve anything (unless the inpatient staff, coming to the situation for the first time, recognise something important that has previously gone unrecognised). Once patients have been admitted because treatment in the community has failed, it is very difficult to discharge them again if they continue to fail to improve (as is often the case). Such situations can drift on for months, with a cycle of second opinions and tertiary referrals that mostly lead nowhere.

Even when admissions have not been prompted by therapeutic frustration, a similar process can develop if there is no provision in the plan for the possibility that the standard treatment might fail. The team then has to improvise, and try to work out what to do next. This is a form of reactive treatment. It is possible and desirable early in most admissions to take into account the possibility that an initial plan will fail, and to have a plan B (and sometimes C and D) in anticipation of this. Similarly, the plan needs to include clarity over the degree of change that is expected. The threshold for discharge is then apparent, and the likely components of the subsequent package of care at home can be anticipated. This allows the team to trace the trajectory of changes in the patient's condition towards an identifiable goal, so that the next steps can be introduced in a timely fashion.

The final common and avoidable cause of overextended admissions is a neglect of continuing problems in the patient's life. For example, if a patient has serious financial problems or is homeless, then waiting until he is 'ready for discharge' before offering him any help with these matters is bound to cause problems. It is inevitable that this will delay or severely complicate discharge and undermine the patient's well being. Help with these types of problems needs to be available early in an admission. Such difficulties are usually evident at the outset. Clinicians also have to identify contextual problems that are likely to develop whilst the patient is in hospital, in order to avoid patients facing difficulties on discharge that are worse than at the time of admission. For example, if someone has rent arrears and no one attends to the problem, arrears continue to accumulate and may reach the point where eviction proceedings commence. The patient may move from financial distress to actual homelessness.

Rapid readmission is a problem that has some features in common with overextended admissions. Indeed, it can be caused by long admissions, whereby the patient becomes dependent on the inpatient environment, struggles to cope on discharge and then wants to return to the hospital. Unresolved social problems can have a similar impact. However, we have to say that the reasons for rapid readmission can be difficult to understand. Rapid relapse and readmission can occur completely without warning or obvious explanation. We suspect that anxiety is a factor that is often overlooked as a cause of deterioration on discharge. Many patients, having recovered from a major episode of serious illness, suffer from quite serious and persistent anxiety after the resolution of more dramatic psychotic or depressive symptoms. There is a tendency to perceive anxiety as a residual and trivial symptom that will resolve of its own accord once the patient gets out of hospital. This may be true, but when anxiety is unchanged or worsens during periods of home leave, it appears to us to predict relapse on discharge. Whilst we know of no empirical evidence to support this assertion, nonetheless we believe it is sensible to offer patients specific treatment for this type of residual anxiety, which normally means some form of behavioural anxiety management.

Rapid readmission is regarded as an objective sign of poor quality of care in the NHS. Mental health services collect data on the ninety-day readmission rate, and a high rate is a key indicator of poor performance. Whilst the reasoning behind this is understandable, not all rapid readmissions represent a serious failure. For example, when patients have complex problems, it is often necessary to employ some creativity in planning discharge and ongoing treatment. It is the nature of things that it is impossible to know whether such plans will work without giving them a try. Discharge planning has to include a willingness to sometimes readmit the patient if things are not working well. This allows for creative thinking without compromising safety.

Main points in this chapter

1. Community treatment includes periods of inpatient care for some patients.
2. Inpatient care is rarely constructive if it is regarded as either the centrepiece of treatment or the default option in the context of treatment failure.
3. Inpatient care has intrinsic problems for patients, especially with regard to loss of freedom and autonomy. Inpatient environments are improved by attention to physical structure and nursing care rather than intrusive security and inflexible programmes of 'therapy'.
4. Inpatient episodes need to follow plans that fit in with longer term treatment strategies. This is facilitated by the involvement of community staff in inpatient treatment planning.
5. The course and structure of inpatient treatment is best planned at the outset, with attention to ongoing problems in the patient's social environment.

8 Compulsion and locked doors

Controversy continues to rage over the use of legal compulsion in the treatment of people suffering from mental illness. The current focus of conflict is over the use of compulsory treatment orders in the community, which already exist in some countries. There has been a long-standing governmental aspiration to introduce them in the UK, and this is likely to happen in the near future. We do not propose to explore the controversy here. Suffice to say that the debate within the mental health community regarding compulsion in general centres on the tension between two positions: What is the point of symptom relief if the price is loss of personal freedom? and What is the point of personal freedom if the consequence is severe mental illness and distress?

The limited use of compulsion is a feature of mental health care in all developed countries, and most mental health professionals recognise that it is sometimes necessary and appropriate. However, few of us are comfortable with the use of compulsion. This unease tends to worsen the longer you practise, as the certainties of youth dissolve into the ambiguities of experience. Few psychiatrists can escape the salutary experience of recommending that a patient should be detained, only to find that other authorised professionals disagree and that the subsequent treatment plan works well, whilst avoiding compulsion. We have written elsewhere about the experience of being detained (Poole & Higgo, 2006). No matter how well intentioned professionals are in the execution of legal compulsion, it is always frightening and frustrating for the patient. It inescapably involves breaking the patient's will, and it can break the patient's spirit. These aspects of compulsion are unequivocally counter-therapeutic, and these are good reasons for being circumspect in exercising legal powers. What is surprising is how forgiving patients can be about detentions, even when they happen repeatedly. However, it would be a mistake to imagine that the fact of detention simply disappears from the therapeutic relationship once the patient has his freedom restored and the dialogue between patient and professional becomes more cordial and civilised. The power relationship is forever skewed, and trust has to be regained through positive effort.

The use of compulsion involves a series of ethical and clinical dilemmas that cannot be resolved by application of a straightforward set of invariable fundamental principles. There are serious adverse consequences in both the overuse and underuse of compulsion. Overuse leads to an authoritarian, paternalistic style of practice that, at its worst, is oppressive and damaging to patients' well being through overzealousness. Underuse leads to an indecisive, pseudo-liberal style of practice that, at its worst, is self-indulgent and damaging to patients' well being through neglect. One routinely encounters situations where it is hard to know if one is falling into these pitfalls. Box 8.1 illustrates the two sides of the dilemma.

We regret to say that there are no easy answers to the ambiguities in the role of compulsion and that, in our opinion, each decision in this regard has to be made in the awareness that both low and high thresholds for using legal powers carry hazards for patients.

Long-term detention

Long-term detention under mental health legislation creates a further set of dilemmas without simple resolution. There is a small but significant group of people who suffer from severe mental illness and who do not respond well to standard treatments. They are, in one way or another, continuously at risk. They are legally detained for long periods, sometimes for decades, and are resident in high-, medium- and low-security psychiatric facilities that are invariably far from their homes. Almost all such care is funded by the state, but more than half of these beds are in the private sector. This pattern of care evolved largely in the absence of any planning. It has been described as 'the virtual asylum' (Poole *et al.*, 2002) in the belief that it has unwittingly replicated several of the shortcomings of the old asylum system. In particular, there is no clear route for patients out of these institutions, and movement back into the community is frustrated by the lack of an appropriate diversity of supported accommodation that can meet individual needs for continuing rehabilitation.

For these patients, long-term compulsion seems unavoidable, in the interests of safety and because the alternative appears to be neglect. However, long-term compulsion is counter-productive in the struggle towards an ordinary existence in the community. Long-term detention is bound to create a secondary handicap of institutionalisation, and rehabilitation then has to focus on overcoming problems caused by the treatment environment. When people make progress, it occurs in the context of a powerful external locus of control. Consequently, it is very hard to know whether this progress will endure in less restrictive settings or whether it is contingent upon compulsion.

The obstructions to providing good-quality, long-term rehabilitation to these forgotten people are primarily due to the prevailing organisation and funding of mental health care. This is highly frustrating, because there are evidence-based rehabilitation approaches that would be more effective and cheaper than the present arrangements. However, the main issue for the ordinary community psychiatrist is that such patients tend to be disowned by their local service of origin, not least because they are out of sight and out of mind. The attitudes of psychiatrists and CMHTs (largely to the effect 'not our problem') can be one of the biggest obstructions to the rehabilitation of these patients. Some community teams have a policy of remaining in close contact with such patients. They review the patients' progress on a regular basis, even when the prospect of a return to the community seems remote. We would suggest that it is an

Box 8.1 Two ways of being wrong over legal compulsion

1. Claire

Claire was in her second year at medical school when she started to notice that other students did not seem to like her. They made tangential remarks about her clothes and her sexuality. They seemed to constantly talk about her. She was distressed, but she was determined not to allow her tormentors to see that she was affected. Her academic performance, which had always been excellent, deteriorated and she failed a series of exams. She was called to see the dean of the faculty, who tried to understand why an able student was struggling. He made little progress, so he explained to her that the General Medical Council (GMC) expected doctors to attend to their own health. He wanted her to see her GP. Under the pressure of a stressful interview, Claire suddenly realised that her peers were acting under the direction of the GMC, and that the dean had been replaced by a GMC assessor. She quit medical school the next day.

Back home with her parents Claire was suffering from acute schizophrenia with Capgras delusions. She talked quite freely about her ideas, but she attended to her self-care and maintained a well-preserved social manner. Her mother took her to their GP, who recognised the nature of the problem and arranged for assessment by the local CMHT. When seen at home, Claire resisted attempts to get her to talk about her ideas, because she believed that the team had been sent by the GMC. She refused to contemplate any form of treatment. Her parents were worried, but they were keen to accept the advice of the professionals. The consultant psychiatrist told them that she was suffering from schizophrenia, but in the light of her well-preserved manner and the lack of any evidence of risk of aggression, self-harm or self-neglect, he was reluctant to use compulsion. He decided to wait and see what happened next.

So things continued over the next ten years. Claire lost contact with her friends, and attempts to work as a secretarial temp failed owing to her lack of concentration. She lived a narrow and limited life at home with her parents, preoccupied with her paranoid beliefs and psychotic experiences. From time to time she would become anxious and agitated, and this led to further psychiatric assessments. As there was little objective change in the situation, there was a continuing strategy of 'wait and see'.

On her thirtieth birthday Claire became very angry that she had never had a boyfriend, had no prospect of having a family and had no career, all because of the GMC. She went to the local police station to complain. The police officers recognised that she was ill, and a series of events ensued that resulted in her being admitted to hospital under the Mental Health Act. There she was treated for the first time, and made a rapid improvement. She gained no insight, but the psychosis abated and she formed a good relationship with the CMHT. Soon after discharge she enrolled for a degree course, she made friends and her quality of life improved beyond recognition. The psychiatrist reproached himself for failing to take more decisive action from the outset. He had known that she was suffering from an illness that was unlikely to resolve without treatment, and his strategy of waiting for things to deteriorate had led to Claire effectively losing ten years of her life.

2. David

David was a thirty-five-year-old man who had suffered from schizophrenia since his late teens. He had always been overindulged by his mother, and his personality was grossly immature. He had used drugs since his early teens, and had a strong preference for amphetamine and cocaine, the effects of which he moderated with heroin. His dominant strategy for dealing with difficulties in life was to become threatening, which was effective because he was tall and thickset. However, he had no history of actual violence. He funded his drug use through begging from his mother and through non-repayable 'loans' from friends. His illness followed an unstable course, and staff did not like nursing him because when he was in hospital he was intimidating.

A crisis arose as a consequence of a noisy argument at David's flat involving some drug-using friends. Neighbours called the police, who charged David with possession of drugs and with allowing the premises to be used for drug dealing. In due course he was convicted, and soon after he was sent an eviction notice because the offences placed him in breach of his tenancy agreement. Under the stress of these events he discontinued antipsychotic medication and his mental state started to deteriorate. On the day of the eviction the consultant psychiatrist, a community mental health nurse and a social worker went round to see him. The psychiatrist was confronted with a chronically antisocial man suffering from a deteriorating psychosis. He was about to become homeless and he was in any case effectively unhousable. The psychiatrist felt that the only sensible strategy was to admit him to hospital under compulsion. The social worker and the nurse disagreed, as did David's GP when he was summoned to the scene. They argued that whilst David was unquestionably antisocial, this was true whether he was acutely mentally ill or not. They suggested that the psychiatrist was really proposing to use legal compulsion to resolve a housing crisis, not a clinical crisis. The psychiatrist felt that this was a rationalisation of a reluctance to admit, because David could be unpleasant.

The psychiatrist had no alternative but to go along with the majority view. David was found accommodation in a bed and breakfast establishment, where he was visited the next morning by the CMHT. The psychiatrist suggested that, if David wanted to resolve his problems, he should accept depot medication. David had always refused this in the past, so everyone was surprised when he accepted the plan. The psychiatrist was even more surprised over the subsequent months to find that David assiduously and uncomplainingly attended for his depot every fortnight. He continued his usual chaotic, antisocial, drug misusing lifestyle, but his mental state stabilised. Two years later, he was still out of hospital, which was his longest unbroken spell in the community since his teens. The psychiatrist had to acknowledge that, despite his suspicions over their motives, the other professionals had been right and he had been wrong.

intrinsic responsibility of CMHTs, including psychiatrists, to take some responsibility for the long-term well being of the most disadvantaged group of people with mental illness.

Locked doors

The development of psychiatry in the UK in the second half of the twentieth century was characterised by an increasing rejection of the use of physical restraint and locked doors. By 1980 there was considerable pride amongst British psychiatrists that physical restraint had been eliminated, in contrast to other European countries. Strapping patients to the bed and the use of straitjackets were seen as atavistic habits of foreigners. This ignored the fact that, at that time, British psychiatrists habitually prescribed disturbed patients medication in doses that were by international standards very high, and that modern psychopharmacologists would regard as positively toxic.

Whilst some aspects of the British 'liberal' approach to inpatient care were based more on conceit than reality, it did lead to a situation that eliminated some of the more obviously oppressive and brutal aspects of asylum treatment. Inpatient environments improved under the assumption that inpatients should be nursed in open conditions unless there was a good reason not to. It is easier for people to accept inpatient treatment if it appears that they can come and go at will, and if the doors are unlocked. No adult can really feel comfortable in a setting where they are locked in and have no access to a key.

The climate of opinion changed sharply from around 1990, with increasing public concern for the safety (or safeness) of people with mental illness. Since that time, locked doors have returned with a vengeance. Security and control of movement in and out of psychiatric units are far more obtrusive than they have been for decades. This is often justified on the grounds that one of the purposes is to keep undesirables out (for example, drug dealers) rather than keeping the patients in, but the purpose of ostentatious security does not alter its effect. If voluntary or informal treatment occurs behind locked doors, then the difference between being detained or not is subtle. Under these conditions, most of the drawbacks of detention affect all patients, detained or otherwise (it is arguable that the detained patients are better off under these circumstances, as they have legal rights and safeguards that do not apply to others). Even the right to refuse treatment is undermined if everyone is locked in, as the shift from choice to compulsion only involves paperwork. If security is intended to improve the therapeutic environment, it is bound to fail as, even when it is necessary, it has counter-therapeutic effects.

Control of movement in and out of inpatient units can be achieved without the use of locked doors, and security does not have to be ostentatious to be effective. It is usually necessary to be firm with people in order to exercise the powers granted to staff under legal compulsion, but firmness does not depend upon oppressive paraphernalia. Locked doors are definitely necessary under some circumstances, and not just in forensic settings. However, they are no substitute for well-designed treatment environments and good-quality nursing care.

PICUs

It has become an item of faith that all inpatient units should include a psychiatric intensive care unit or PICU. These are small, locked wards with a high staff-to-patient ratio. There is little or no empirical evidence on the need for, or effects of, PICUs. We worked for many years in a service where there was no PICU. Although there was some controversy over this, there was no evidence that it had adverse consequences in terms of referrals to forensic units, abscond rates, violent incidents or harm to either patients or the public (as compared with similar areas that did have a PICU). The situation changed because the expense of close nursing of disturbed patients on an open unit was regarded as prohibitive.

Herein lies our first reservation about PICUs. There is always a suspicion that locked wards are used as a means to reduce the nursing costs of open wards. Our other concerns are:

• If PICU beds exist, they will be used. If there is a four-bed PICU it will always contain the four most disturbed patients on the unit rather than solely being reserved for those who objectively 'need' this form of care.

• PICUs rarely offer a good therapeutic environment. Once the most disturbed and distressed patients have been placed together, they overstimulate and frighten each other, creating a vicious cycle of disturbance.

• PICUs deskill the rest of the staff in managing acute disturbance. As some patients become disturbed unexpectedly, this deskilling may compromise the safety and quality of overall patient care.

• Some patients, such as young black men, may be perceived as particularly threatening. Decisions to nurse patients in PICUs are vulnerable to this kind of stereotyping, which, over time, has an impact in alienating parts of the community from the mental health services.

• Many PICUs offer little in the way of intensive care, and are simply custodial 'lockups'. They may be used to simply prevent patients from absconding, which is entirely inappropriate.

Our skepticism about the value of PICUs will not make them disappear, and they are likely to be a feature of inpatient treatment for the foreseeable future. We do believe that it is possible to use a PICU constructively, but only if there is a high level of awareness of the potential pitfalls.

At the end of the day, we have to live with it

Despite the many worrying aspects of the use of compulsion and security in psychiatric treatment, we believe that the complete rejection of them can only be advocated by either denying the fundamental nature of some mental illnesses or by an irresponsible disregard for the serious consequences for some mentally ill people if they were abolished. Mental health professionals have to accept and own these aspects of treatment, because to do otherwise is dishonest. If we distance ourselves from one necessary aspect of treatment, then the whole package of care becomes disjointed and less effective, and the plight of those who are under compulsion or locked up worsens, rather than improves. Whilst there may be no full resolution to the problems of detention, some of the problems can be ameliorated by the recognition that high-quality care is more important than reinforced steel doors.

Main points in this chapter

1. The use of legal compulsion and locked doors are, under some circumstances, an unavoidable part of mental health treatment.
2. The use of these measures has a tangible negative impact on patients, and the effect on therapeutic relationships persists long after compulsion ceases.
3. There is a group of people who experience long-term detention in remote facilities. Mental health professionals can obstruct these patients' recovery if they disown them.
4. Safe and secure environments for the treatment of detained patients can be achieved through well-planned and skilled nursing care and well-designed treatment environments. An oppressive paraphernalia of security may have an adverse impact on all patients, not just those who are detained.

9   Not at home, not in hospital

Even enthusiastic community psychiatrists have to acknowledge that some people with mental health problems cannot and should not be treated either in their own home or in hospital. The predominant international model of psychiatric practice is office-based one-to-one treatment. There is a large literature concerning this therapeutic environment. We would not suggest that there is anything intrinsically wrong with practising in this way. However, there are some problems associated with the main 'not at home, not in hospital' treatment options as they have developed in the UK. Traditional practices require modification if they are to continue to play a functional role in newer models of service provision, and some modalities of treatment may have to be abandoned all together.

The main problems associated with UK patterns of mental health practice have arisen because service development has tended to occur on an ad hoc basis. New approaches have been grafted onto traditional ways of working. In all fields of human endeavour, the familiar tends to be comfortable, which is why traditional ways of doing things sometimes persist long after they have become outmoded and dysfunctional. In Britain, as in many other countries, modern psychiatry developed out of the treatment of severely ill people in large mental hospitals. After the Second World War, psychiatrists started to practise beyond the asylum walls. As they did so, they extended the range of conditions that they attempted to treat. This coincided with the formation of the National Health Service, and the provision of comprehensive state-funded health care. The development of psychiatric outpatient clinics was an important step towards non-institutional care. Clinics were established following the model of general medical outpatient clinics. Alongside this, day hospitals emerged from the 1950s as a type of intermediate care, based on the rationale that patients did not need to be in hospital twenty-four hours a day in order to receive treatment. It was another important step towards community mental health care (Freeman, 2005).

This configuration of inpatient, outpatient and day hospital care was the backbone of mental health services over several decades. Despite the accelerating change in practice over the last fifteen years, some UK services continue to adhere to this pattern of treatment as the main focus of their activity, with community teams operating alongside them in an uncomfortable parallel co-existence.

Outpatient clinics

British psychiatry has a strong attachment to genericism. This has not been broken by central government policies that favour multiple specialist teams and that prioritise the treatment of people suffering from severe and enduring mental illness. Consequently, most British general adult psychiatrists work with people suffering from a wide variety of mental health problems. Many psychiatrists continue to have most of their contact with patients in outpatient clinics.

Traditional British outpatient clinics are usually conducted on hospital sites in dedicated office suites. The premises have rarely been designed for this purpose, and often have been inherited by mental health services after they have been abandoned as unsuitable by other medical specialities. Premises are usually of an inadequate size to comfortably accommodate the number of staff and patients that use them in the course of the working day. Décor and ambience are low priorities in financially stretched state services, and redecoration cycles are too long to maintain acceptable standards. This creates a sadly familiar style of interior design which is soulless and shabby. Standards of construction are often poor, so that privacy is compromised by sound penetration through doors and walls.

New patients are offered one-hour assessment appointments. Follow-up appointments are for fifteen minutes. A typical follow-up clinic includes a group of patients suffering from schizophrenia or bipolar affective disorder who have been attending for years or decades. They are often seen by an unending succession of junior psychiatrists in training. There is another group of patients who are being followed up after a crisis admission, and yet another group suffering from anxiety, depression and other moderately severe mental disorders who have been referred by their family doctors. The latter two groups show a degree of turnover, with patients attending every four to six weeks for a few months or years. Receptionists, psychiatrists and patients tend to struggle with the problems that are set out in Box 9.1. These are so common and so difficult to eradicate that we have reached the conclusion that they are intrinsic to this style of working, and they have to be regarded as physical laws.

We had much of our training in these clinics, and we worked in this way through our early years as consultants. From about 1990 we were based in CMHTs. Teams came to regard medical time as a resource that was in short supply. They knew that we were spending about a third of our time in clinic and they started to ask us what we were achieving with patients when they attended. As they failed to get a satisfactory answer to this question, they started to ask still more pointed questions about the general purpose of the clinics.

It was at this point that we realised that we did not really know why we were seeing patients in clinic. Eventually, following painful reflection, we came to realise that the combination of a lack of clear objectives and the intrinsic problems of the style of working meant that everybody involved had been wasting a great deal of time. This was not a unique insight. The same debate was happening in many teams across the country. It turned out that there was a better way of doing things, whereby the same number of professionals saw the same number of patients, but everyone was considerably happier with the treatment process. This culminated in a national initiative, 'New Ways of Working' (Department of Health, 2005), aimed at promoting alternative patterns of practice. Box 9.2 sets out one way of reorganising psychiatrists' outpatient work within a multidisciplinary team. It does not describe all of the implications of these

Box 9.1 Eleven immutable features of the traditional British outpatient clinic

1. *Outpatient clinics are always fully booked up for at least the next three months.* Many patients need to be seen more frequently than this, and some people need to be seen urgently. Consequently, appointments have to be double booked. If overbooking is resolved by opening a further clinic session, this rapidly becomes overbooked too.
2. *Patients are never seen at the right appointment time.* This is a consequence of short appointments and double bookings. Patients have to sit for long periods in crowded waiting rooms. This makes many of them anxious, which then makes the interview more difficult.
3. *Clinics are conducted with a constant sense of time urgency.* Even where the psychiatrist is skilled at concealing his own sense of urgency, many patients realise that the clinic is busy, so they try to help by keeping things brief. The psychiatrist then fails to get a clear picture of the patient's current situation.
4. *There is not enough time for the psychiatrist to do much more than find out how the patient is doing and alter their medication.* Most patients need more than just medication, but non-pharmacological interventions have to be carried out by someone else or not at all.
5. *Team members have to protect the patient from the psychiatrist.* The psychiatrist is often unable to obtain a proper understanding of the patient's situation in the time available and has to make decisions in isolation from other team members. Other professionals attend with the patient in order to prevent the psychiatrist from making bad decisions, which is a waste of their time. There are better ways to make joint assessments and plans.
6. *Clinics can only ever be too busy or too quiet.* Not surprisingly, many patients do not like these clinics. Consequently there is a high rate of non-attendance (as opposed to cancellation of appointments). Because of the way that booking systems are organised, appointments for patients who are unlikely to turn up aggregate on particular days. There is never a happy medium. Whilst busy clinics are often exhausting, quiet ones can be stultifyingly boring. Although psychiatrists often believe that their clinics are only workable because a lot of patients do not attend, actually non-attendances increase pressure on clinic time.
7. *Holidays are a source of anxiety and pressure for the psychiatrist.* In the run up to leave, there is a crescendo of demand on clinic time, and the psychiatrist goes on holiday in a state of nervous exhaustion that resolves about two days before he returns to work.
8. *Patients are never discharged, they are only ever lost to follow-up.* Because there is no clarity regarding reasons for attendance, it is difficult for either doctor or patient to recognise that discharge is appropriate. Some patients politely continue to attend indefinitely. Others get fed up and stop coming. Few have a planned discharge.

9. *A 'good' appointment is one where the patient is OK and there is little for the psychiatrist to do.* One might suppose that psychiatrists are most effective when they deploy their clinical skills. However, this takes time. Most doctors in these clinics are relieved if there is little to do and they can move on to the next patient.

10. *Clinics can only be closed in their entirety.* Closing one clinic session each week throws intolerable pressure on the remaining clinic sessions. Consequently, clinic time can only ever be increased, never reduced. It is, however, easier than one might suppose to stop doing clinics completely and to find other ways of delivering treatment.

11. *Despite all of the above, most psychiatrists like holding clinics.* Many patients gradually become old friends, and it is genuinely nice to see them, especially if they are well. This is one of the reasons that psychiatrists resist changing their practices. However, although doctor and patient might enjoy chatting, this is not a legitimate purpose for a clinic. 'Goodbye, you are discharged' has far greater therapeutic potency. Psychiatrists should be encouraged to find a proper social life of their own.

working patterns, but it does illustrate that there are safe and efficient alternatives to clinics.

We have not abandoned one-to-one office-based psychiatric treatment in totality. We continue to see small numbers of patients in this setting. The real point here is that it is perfectly possible to work very hard but rather ineffectively, especially if you lack clarity as to the purpose of treatment. There are often unexpected benefits from thinking seriously about aspects of your practice that you had previously taken for granted. In reviewing the purpose of outpatient clinics we came to realise that it is important to think about the purpose of each interaction with a patient beforehand, to be clear about what one is trying to achieve at that particular interview, and to be clear how this forms part of a strategy to attain overall treatment objectives. One of the frequently raised objections to the abandonment of clinics is that they are time efficient. However, our experience is to the contrary. Smaller numbers of more focussed interviews are more effective and more time efficient. Having relinquished outpatient clinics with some reluctance, we prefer this new style of working.

The evidence for the overall superiority of community treatment seems strong, but it does have some real disadvantages. Treating people in their own homes is a departure from normal medical practice. It can create problems in maintaining boundaries and in protecting confidentiality. Some people find it intrusive. Following from this, office-based outpatient treatment is the location of choice when:

- the patient has a strong preference in the matter;
- home circumstances make privacy and confidentiality difficult (for example, when the patient lives in a communal setting);
- boundary issues are particularly important, as can be the case with some psychological treatments and when treating people with some types of personality problems;

Box 9.2 An alternative to the outpatient clinic in multidisciplinary teams

1. New referrals come to the team, not the doctor. A screening assessment is carried out, which only involves one of the doctors if it is obvious from the outset that there is a significant medical issue to be tackled.
2. Patients with active treatment plans are reviewed by the doctor with their key worker, either at home or at the office. Routine reviews for strategic treatment planning may occur as infrequently as once a year. Joint interviews are also organised to resolve particular problems as they arise. They can be arranged at short notice in order to deal with urgent problems.
3. Patients with no active treatment plan are discharged to their GP, but given easy access to rapid intervention from the team at their own or other people's request.
4. Doctors take a role in one-to-one treatment where they have particular and relevant skills, aimed at achieving specific objectives.
5. These measures eliminate routine appointments with the psychiatrist to check how the patient is doing and non-attendance rates drop dramatically. This saves a lot of time. It allows the psychiatrist to focus on specific and relevant problems, and makes him more available for urgent interventions.

- the problem is not severe and the treatment plan only demands the involvement of one professional;
- the patient represents a threat to visiting professionals;
- the patient is in the process of recovering and wants to move away from an obviously 'mental health' pattern of service and towards a less intensive relationship with the team.

Clearly, the proportion of patients falling into these categories varies according to the demography of the area and the purpose of the team, so that it is difficult to determine an optimum level of residual clinic activity. However, brief outpatient appointments seem to us to be a waste of time, even in the listed circumstances. We suggest that half-hour appointments are usually optimal in community psychiatry practice. If there is insufficient material to usefully discuss with the patient for half an hour, one has to question whether the patient needs to be seen at all.

In all forms of community mental health work there is a need to hold meetings from time to time with patients and their families, sometimes with a number of professionals in attendance. These meetings are difficult to conduct in the average-sized office or, for that matter, the average-sized house. Meeting rooms in the CMHT base are the most appropriate setting for these meetings. We have found that patients and their families tend to like the format where everyone sits around a large table, partially for practical reasons concerning the need to fill in forms, but also, we think, because of the levelling effect of a round (or square) table discussion. The setting seems to feel more businesslike and does not clearly belong to the doctor in the way that his office docs.

The strange rise and fall of the day hospital

The implicit rationale for day hospitals (where patients could safely sleep at home, it was less disruptive to their lives to have them attend hospital only for active interventions) made sense, and they spread widely. Until recently they were regarded as an intrinsic component of a comprehensive mental health service, and every British service had a day hospital of some sort. At their inception, they offered most of the treatments that were available to inpatients, including some of the more dramatic contemporary treatments such as electroconvulsive therapy (ECT) and intravenous infusion of antidepressants, but they also offered a range of psychological and diversional interventions (Briscoe *et al.*, 2004). It is disappointing to report that over the whole of our working lifetimes there has been a sense that day hospitals often (or perhaps usually) become dysfunctional. The focus for discontent has tended to be that they drift away from the treatment of severe mental illness, and towards the treatment of less severe disorders. Furthermore, patients tend to attend for long periods, often years. Day hospitals appear to have retained some of the problematic features of full hospitalisation, especially decontextualisation of problems and the promotion of dependency.

There were repetitive attempts to refocus day hospitals on the treatment of people with severe and acute mental illness. Despite this, they persistently attracted two main groups of people. The first group consisted of people suffering from psychotic illness who had difficulty in accessing ordinary social activities. This was a legitimate function, particularly where it was part of an overall rehabilitation plan aimed at restoring a normal social life. However, it did not require the involvement of a full hospital staff group. This function has been taken over by non-hospital day services that are increasingly provided by the voluntary sector. The second group consisted of people suffering from chronic anxiety and depression. For these people, the dependency promoting qualities of hospital settings were damaging. Long-term attendance rarely led to much change, and the ability to avoid problems in a supportive setting could make things worse, not better.

A few years ago, following a strong policy initiative to target mental health services at the most severely ill patients, day hospitals were re-branded as 'partial hospitalisation' services. The concept was to provide intensive treatment to acutely ill patients as an alternative to hospital admission (Priebe *et al.*, 2006). However, partial hospitalisation lacked the key feature of inpatient admission, namely control. This meant, for example, that there was no way of preventing heavy drinking or drug misuse from complicating the treatment of severely unwell and disinhibited patients. Whilst this is commonly a problem during inpatient admissions, it can be contained more easily in that setting. Attempts to treat patients suffering from mania through partial hospitalisation were particularly liable to failure. Some patients, such as those suffering from relapses of schizophrenia, did recover well during partial hospitalisation, but it became increasingly evident that they usually did equally well when treated in their own homes.

Once disillusionment with partial hospitalisation became widespread, mental health day hospitals started to close down. This process is now quite advanced, and there appears to be a growing belief that day services are not generally useful and that the staff are better deployed in other, newer roles. We believe that this assessment is correct. However, there are presently some promising small-scale experiments based on the day hospital model, where specialised interventions are offered to people with specific problems such as recurrent deliberate self-harm or borderline personality disorder. It is too soon to know if these approaches will prove successful and gain general acceptance. Overall, it seems safe to state that the concept of the day hospital as a key component to general mental health services is dead.

Treating people in unusual settings

Some mentally ill people live in unusual environments, the key examples being single homeless people and prisoners. Many of us have a paternalistic or philanthropic urge to 'rescue' such people by admitting them to hospital. Although this is sometimes the right thing to do, it can be naive and unproductive. Homelessness is part of a constellation of disadvantage. Single homeless people do not suffer from a simple lack of housing, but tend to follow a pattern of unstable accommodation, punctuated by brief periods of rooflessness. They tend to be people who have deep seated difficulties due to emotionally deprived or abusive childhoods with inconsistent or absent parenting. They often have ingrained behaviours that make them hard to tolerate as neighbours or co-habitees. They frequently have problems with substance dependency. Many of them support themselves through sex work. They have recurrent contact with police and criminal justice agencies both as perpetrators and victims of crime.

Homeless people have surprisingly supportive (if deviant) social networks. They utilise facilities such as soup kitchens and homelessness day centres that are beyond the awareness of the settled community. When homeless people are mentally unwell, the obvious thing to do is to admit them to hospital, treat their illness, and rehouse them. Whilst this is sometimes successful, more often it is followed by a return to the streets and their habitual chaotic lifestyle. Their mental illness then relapses. What really offends liberal sensibilities is that many homeless people prefer to live in that setting. They are unable to cope with a settled existence and they find the homeless lifestyle supportive and undemanding.

Many homeless people with mental illness are better treated in their own chaotic setting. This takes a great deal of skill and specialised knowledge of their way of life and the broader 'homeless community'. With patience and persistence it is possible to treat them in their own environment. Small, slow steps can eventually lead to change and resettlement. Progress in this manner can lead to a much more robust and constructive change than is possible by means of a more dramatic 'rescue'.

Similarly, the problem with admitting prisoners to hospital is that they often have to go back to prison once they are better. A recovery that is contingent on the hospital setting is unlikely to persist on return to prison. Furthermore, many long-term prisoners find the prison environment less stressful than either ordinary life or secure hospital settings. We do not suggest that prisoners should never be transferred to hospital for treatment. However, just as is the case for some homeless people, some prisoners are more likely to get better and stay better if they are treated in living circumstances that are, for them, familiar and supportive.

Quite apart from the fact that working with such patients requires specialist skills and knowledge, it also requires the ability to compromise on a range of issues concerning clinical practice. This can take the mental health professional to the absolute limit of what is professionally and ethically acceptable. Without vigilance, it is easy to cross the boundary into the unacceptable. There are frequently dilemmas that defy simple resolution. For example:

- The only opportunity to interview a psychotic homeless man may be at a soup kitchen crowded with other homeless people. Neither his dignity nor his confidentiality can be preserved under these circumstances, but the alternative is to make no assessment at all. Does he have any less right to confidentiality and dignity than anyone else, or do his peculiar circumstances mean that the interests of his mental health come before all else?
- Mental health professionals may only be allowed into prisons on condition that they observe prison rules. These may place very difficult demands on the clinician. They may dictate that, if the prisoner discloses that they are currently using drugs, this information should be passed to the prison authorities. The prisoner/patient will then be punished. Should the professional break confidentiality? Should he undertake to follow prison regulations at all, given that he will be refused entry if he declines to do so?
- Tobacco is an important commodity amongst prisoners and the homeless. Offering a suspicious homeless person or prisoner a cigarette is a culturally congruent and effective way of establishing an initial contact. Is it acceptable for a health professional to promote a lethal addiction just because it is expedient to do so?

Threats to boundaries and compromises of acceptable professional behaviour arise constantly when treating people in such unusual settings. However, these marginalised people are severely disadvantaged. Conventional approaches to treatment routinely fail them. In our opinion, it is so important to help these people to secure meaningful treatment that it is worth grappling with the ambiguities of a professional life at the outer edge of respectable practice.

Main points in this chapter

1. Traditional psychiatric outpatient clinics do not work well as part of modern multi-disciplinary team working.
2. Office-based one-to-one psychiatric treatment does have a continuing role as part of the range of mental health interventions. It is the modality of choice for the treatment of people suffering with some particular types of mental health problems.
3. Day hospitals seemed like a good idea, but have a very limited role in modern community psychiatry.

4. Some people have lifestyles that make conventional patterns of care inappropriate and ineffective. It is possible for mental health professionals to enter these patients' environments and thus make effective interventions. This work requires specialist knowledge and skills. It constantly generates problems over boundaries and professional behaviour that cannot easily be resolved, which have to remain in clinicians' awareness if they are to avoid drifting into unacceptable practice.

10   Models of care

We believe that the success of psychiatric treatment depends upon the quality of therapeutic relationships between mental health professionals and patients. This is not necessarily self-evident. Manualised treatments have been developed on the assumption that operationalised manoeuvres are the 'signal' of treatment and that issues concerning the therapeutic relationship are 'noise'. However, our understanding of the evidence, both scientific and experiential, suggests that the relationship between professional and patient is a critical factor in achieving a good outcome (McCabe & Priebe, 2004).

It seems to us that effective mental health professionals develop personal skills that allow specific treatments to facilitate patients' recovery from mental illness. These skills concern the application of scientific knowledge to complex clinical situations and the management of therapeutic relationships. Weak or ineffective professionals lack these skills, so that they struggle to construct rational and coherent treatment plans, or their therapeutic relationships with patients are of a poor quality. When weak clinicians use the same specific treatments as their more skilled colleagues, the outcome of treatment tends to be not as good.

Therapeutic relationships are profoundly influenced by the context in which they arise. The configuration of a team, and one's position within it, has a major effect on the nature of individual therapeutic relationships. Junior professionals, who have to defer many decisions to senior colleagues, form different types of therapeutic relationships from those formed by autonomous professionals who can be decisive and speak with the authority of experience (although this is not to say that junior professionals are necessarily less effective than their seniors). The social characteristics of the area in which you work have a major impact. Therapeutic relationships with marginalised and poverty stricken people are different to those with the well heeled and well educated.

There is, however, another type of contextual factor that is less obvious but has an equally powerful effect on therapeutic relationships. This is the model of care which you work within. Sometimes this is not explicit. The model of care is frequently taken to be a 'given', too deeply embedded in the structure of everyday work to be critically examined. It is created by a combination of social policy, economics, the attitudes of professionals and prevalent social attitudes towards people with mental illness. These factors create some contradictions. Consequently, at all times in the history of psychiatry there has been more than one available model of care.

Broadly speaking, there are two main models of care prevalent across the world, creating two types of relationships between people suffering from mental illness and the mental health services. They are to some extent contradictory, but in most countries they exist alongside each other. The first type of relationship characterises mental illness as a problem that is associated with a wide variety of other difficulties. It recognises that people with mental illness are often disadvantaged in obtaining help, not just with regard to their mental health, but also with their physical and social well being. They may actively resist intervention. Services are designed to overcome these layers of disadvantage and resistance to seeking help. They take on a high degree of responsibility for their patients' well being, and are hence intrinsically paternalistic. This is the dominant model where state-funded services attempt to provide comprehensive care. In the UK there is a well-established system of care co-ordination for people with serious mental health problems called the Care Programme Approach, which codifies this type of relationship (Department of Health, 1990). We shall call the overall concept the *care programme model*.

The second type of relationship follows the premise that patients actively seek help with discreet identifiable problems. These problems are amenable to resolution through interventions (or sequences of interventions) which follow more or less predictable patterns and have quantifiable benefits and drawbacks. The patient is an autonomous consumer and treatment is a commodity. Patients make informed choices about which treatment to accept from which clinician. The clinician takes responsibility for delivering interventions competently, but the patient retains full responsibility for their overall well being. This is the dominant model where mental health care is provided by professionals who are not state employees. We shall call this type of relationship the *patient-as-consumer model*.

In the UK, although the care programme model remains predominant, the patient-as-consumer model is of increasing importance both in the private sector and the NHS. The care programme model emphasises the vulnerability of people with mental illness. Poor physical health, poor nutrition, unemployment and social isolation are very real problems for a lot of people suffering from serious mental illness. They cannot overcome the effects of mental illness unless they are helped to resolve some of these problems. Special measures to achieve this can be integrated within the care programme model. The care programme model is compatible with assertive outreach, community treatment orders, supported housing and long-term follow-up. However, because it is intrinsically paternalistic, it embraces elements of duress and frequently undermines patients' autonomy. Patients can experience services based on this model as intrusive, oppressive and marginalising. It is difficult to make meaningful choice a feature of this model, at least with regard to who treats you and in what setting. The care programme model is burdened with the paradox that recovery requires serious effort to overcome a range of adverse effects of receiving this type of care, such as dependency on specialist services and the stigma of being a user of identifiable mental health facilities.

The patient-as-consumer model lends itself to clear care pathways, short-term interventions, measurable treatment outcomes and patient choice. It is difficult to reconcile it with the types of approach that benefit the most vulnerable patients. Indeed, it is at the mercy of Tudor Hart's inverse care law (Tudor Hart, 1971). This states that

---

Box 10.1 Help is at hand

Just before Christmas, a British regional newspaper carried an editorial feature based on an interview with a psychiatrist from a local private psychiatric clinic ('Beating the blues,' *Manchester Evening News*, 21 December 2004). This stated that Christmas is a highly stressful time and that 'clinical stress is a real mental health issue'. There was a description of a range of serious consequences of stress. The psychiatrist was quoted as saying 'if … self-help strategies aren't working, seek professional help'. This was followed by the contact details for the private clinic. The psychiatrist may have been quoted out of context, but the story seemed to invite readers to secure treatment for a short-term and self-limiting problem. We would suggest that anyone seeking help from a psychiatrist solely to assist with the stress associated with Christmas would be making a very poor choice indeed. When mental health intervention is offered to the general public as autonomous consumers, they can be vulnerable to unnecessary intervention.

---

when health care is distributed as a market commodity, resources tend to be directed towards those with the least health need. Tudor Hart asserted that health care could be regarded as a commodity even when most provision was state funded. Because of the close association between severe mental illness and a lack of personal resources, the model carries the risk that the needs of the most vulnerable will be neglected. People whose problems do not fit into a neat category, such as might attract an ICD or DSM coding, can also have difficulty in securing treatment. The other intrinsic weakness of the patient-as-consumer model is that it depends on assumptions that consumers are able to take responsibility for their own well being and that they are in a position to make good choices. However, even the mentally well can be led into making bad choices about mental health treatment (see Box 10.1).

It might appear that a neat way of accommodating these contrasting strengths and weaknesses would be to apply the care programme model to people suffering from psychotic illnesses, and the patient-as-consumer model to people suffering from problems associated with anxiety and depression. Unfortunately, life is not so simple. There are people who unequivocally can be more appropriately helped through one model or the other. However, the majority of patients suffering from the full range of psychiatric diagnoses have needs that shift and change with time depending on the phase of treatment and alterations in their mental state. In the UK, treatment can move back and forth between the two models within a single episode of treatment. This can cause real problems. Patients who have been led to believe that they have choices may find that care programmes can only be delivered by a locality-based service. They then have very little choice over who treats them. Co-ordination of different aspects of care can be difficult and frustrating under the patient-as-consumer model. Patients who have been led to believe that they are going to be offered comprehensive care can be dismayed to find that different aspects of care are provided by different agencies. They can find that agencies have very different attitudes with respect to important issues such as risk and the extent to which service users are expected to resolve their own problems.

Whichever model we work within, clinicians have responsibility for the key task of getting alongside the patient. It is no good to simply rail against the shortcomings of any model or system of care, for they will always exist. If treatment is to be successful, we eventually have to find a way through the ambiguities that are embedded in therapeutic relationships concerning control, duress, independence and autonomy. Finding a route to a truly facilitative relationship is affected by important issues concerning the patient's 'insight', the risks that their mental illness creates for them and their ability to take personal responsibility for their own well being. These issues have an intimate relationship with the developing concept of mental capacity.

Mental capacity

From the very beginning of organised mental health care, both psychiatry and the legal system have been concerned with mental incapacity, meaning impairment of an individual's ability to make informed and considered decisions as a consequence of mental or physical disorder. The legal system has mainly been concerned with mental incapacity with regard to the ability to make decisions about property and financial affairs, personal responsibility for criminality and consent to medical treatment (with separate legal frameworks for mental and physical illness). There are less prominent laws on mental incapacity affecting a variety of other areas such as consent to marriage. All legal systems that are based on British common law (which includes North America) have a well-developed model of mind based on Judeo-Christian theology and moral philosophy. This attaches importance to the exercise of free will in all human affairs. The legal system makes a consequent assumption that people are capable of making their own decisions unless it is clearly demonstrated otherwise.

Psychiatry, on the other hand, has a more ambiguous attitude towards free will. Nearly all scientific models of thought and behaviour, whether these stem from experimental psychology, psychoanalysis or neuroscience, are deterministic. A range of tangible factors is held to affect people's thinking and behaviour and the effect of them is taken to be understandable and predictable. There is little room for free will in these models. However, psychiatry is prone to some inconsistency in this regard, invoking free will in its understanding of certain conditions such as addiction and personality disorder in the guise of the constructs of motivation and volition. This creates a logical inconsistency. We do not intend to explore this here, as it would involve a lengthy philosophical digression, and in any case, we do not have a resolution to it. The practical consequence is that psychiatry has a broad concept of mental incapacity. Mental disorder is understood to have an impact on a wide range of emotional and cognitive functions, with subtle but deleterious effects on patients' ability to make considered judgements. However, this impact is seen as being greater in psychotic and organic disorders than in neurotic and other disorders. This complex approach to the understanding of the psychological concept of judgement underpins the profession's continued recourse to paternalism towards patients.

Despite long-standing concern with mental incapacity, the concept of mental capacity has taken on a new salience that is reflected in the change from talking about *incapacity* to talking about *capacity*. Psychiatry has been increasingly influenced by the service user movement, and has come to take the autonomy of patients much more seriously, both as a value and as an important clinical objective. This has created a new focus on mental capacity as an everyday issue. In the UK there is now a Mental Capacity Act which creates a definition of incapacity and a mechanism for making decisions in people's best interests if they are deemed to lack mental capacity.

In UK law, individuals are not deemed to lack mental capacity as a general personal characteristic. Capacity exists (or does not) with regard to particular decisions at specific moments in time. The law recognises that people have a general right to make eccentric or irrational decisions, even if this leads to consequences that others regard as being against their best interests (e.g. death). There is a three-stage test to assess whether a person has mental capacity with regard to a particular decision. The test can only be applied if (a) the relevant information is given in a form that the person can understand and (b) the person has access to appropriate facilities to allow them to communicate their wishes.

A person lacks capacity if they (a) cannot comprehend the information they are given or (b) cannot retain the information or (c) cannot use and weigh the information to arrive at a decision. In addition to this, there is a group of people who suffer from the rare 'locked in' syndrome. They are paralysed but retain normal cognitive abilities, including full awareness of their surroundings. A small proportion of them cannot communicate, even by blinking. They are deemed to lack capacity because they cannot communicate their wishes.

These principles are laid down in the Mental Capacity Act, but they are based on previous common law principles which were similar. These stated that mental capacity involved comprehension and retention of information, with an ability to weigh the information in the balance. However, the common law principles included a fourth stage to the test. People who were unable to believe salient information were deemed to lack capacity. The question of belief is excluded from the Act, which reflects the legal position that *incapacity* and *irrationality* are not synonymous (or even closely related) in English law.

The UK law with regard to compulsory hospital treatment for mental disorder is set out in the Mental Health Act. Psychiatric treatment under this Act is not affected by the Mental Capacity Act. The Mental Health Act has been undergoing a long and controversial process of revision, and the details of the eventual changes are unclear at the time of writing. The UK law is relevant here only because it illustrates some general principles and paradoxes regarding mental capacity.

The Mental Health Act 1983 introduced a right of appeal for all patients substantively detained. It also introduced a legal requirement for an independent second opinion after three months of treatment in the absence of consent. There had never previously been any independent review of the content of treatment of detained patients. There was no provision in the Mental Health Act 1983 relating to mental capacity, either with respect to criteria for detention or in determining the content of treatment without consent.

In other words, the existence of a serious mental health problem was sufficient to override patients' wishes, irrespective of whether they had a full understanding of their situation (and thus mental capacity) or not.

Work on a new Mental Health Act commenced in about 1999. The advice of a government-appointed expert committee reflected a consensus amongst those involved in mental health services that liability to compulsory treatment should be limited to those who lacked mental capacity. This was logical. If patients understand the consequences of refusing psychiatric treatment, there would appear to be little ethical justification in preventing them from doing so, no matter how unwise this might seem. The government rejected this and other recommendations, leading to persistent conflict with the mental health community and a long delay in legislation.

Bearing in mind that the same government enacted the Mental Capacity Act, there were accusations that policy makers believed that everyone had the right to make unwise or irrational decisions except those who suffer from mental illness. As the freedom to make bad decisions is an intrinsic element of autonomy, this appeared to be an institutional obstruction to the task of helping people progress towards recovery. However, whilst media campaigns over a mythical rising tide of violence by mentally ill people undoubtedly influenced the position of the policy makers, more complex forces probably also had an impact. If public attitudes to the mentally ill are contradictory, so too are some of the attitudes of mental health professionals.

Mental capacity as a clinical concept

The growing concern with mental capacity as a relevant clinical concept is tempered by two other clinical preoccupations, namely *risk* and *insight*. We have noted elsewhere that the concept of insight as a personal attribute is muddled. It makes little sense phenomenologically or psychologically. Insight is really a characteristic of the therapeutic relationship based on whether the clinician and the patient can find sufficient common ground to make progress. Risk is relevant because mental health professionals are concerned with consequences. The judiciary can decide whether someone has the mental capacity to make an evidently disastrous decision. It then moves on to the next case. Mental health professionals have to deal with the aftermath of disastrous decisions. One can make arguments either way as to which of them is better placed to judge the situation. To a psychiatrist, people suffering from a mental disorder may be able to comprehend, retain and weigh information, but they may still suffer from an impairment of the ability to make authentic decisions.

Take the example of a twenty-year-old woman suffering from anorexia nervosa, with a body mass index of twelve. She is close to a degree of weight loss that is incompatible with life. She slips into a metabolic crisis but wants to discharge herself from the medical ward as soon as she has recovered sufficiently to be able to stand up. She accepts that she is underweight and insists that she will try to eat more at home. She insists that she does not want to die. She is told that it is highly unlikely that she will manage to gain weight at home, and that in any case she is at risk of re-feeding syndrome, an unstable metabolic state caused by a rapid change from catabolism to anabolism. She is strongly advised to accept treatment, either in a medical or a psychiatric ward. She prefers to go home and 'do it my way'. She is not suffering from psychosis, dementia or a primary affective disorder. According to the legal criteria she has capacity to make this decision, as she can understand, retain and use the information she is given.

However, people suffering from severe weight loss develop demonstrable cognitive impairments. These are reversible and mostly affect higher executive functions. Starving people can become very concrete in their thinking, with an abnormal focus on immediate or short-term goals. In any case, people with anorexia nervosa have an intense pathological fear of fatness. The salience of this central concern leads them into all manner of bad and life-destroying decisions.

When patients like this are detained and re-fed, the cognitive deficits improve. Sometimes, the underlying anorexic psychopathology changes as well. It is not generally very helpful to detain people with eating disorders, and inpatient care has a very limited role in the treatment of these conditions. However, it seems that people with anorexia can meet the legal criteria for mental capacity with regard to refusal of treatment and yet still have demonstrable and reversible impairments that affect decision making. Similarly, many people with acute schizophrenia may not have a specific impairment that directly affects any of the three elements of legal mental capacity, but the combined effects of thought disorder, overarousal, delusional beliefs and distressing psychotic experiences may make their judgements poor and ill considered.

There are real ambiguities and dilemmas over the extent to which we can legitimately interfere in the lives of people with mental illness, or, to reframe this, the extent to which we should seek to protect them from the consequences of their illness. Perhaps it is not surprising that we cope with this by moving between models of care and have care programme models and patient-as-consumer models running side by side (or alternating during a long-term contact with mental health services). The complete abandonment of medical paternalism is easy to justify as an abstraction and hard to implement. It is very difficult to stand by and watch people run into major problems that might be avoided through the use of paternalistic duress. We have to learn somehow to be aware of, and manage, these shifts in the underlying model of treatment.

Insight and responsibility

The difficulties with the concept of insight do not disappear simply through understanding it as a quality embedded in a therapeutic relationship. It certainly is not a quality that people either possess or lack and, like mental capacity, it is not a general personal attribute. Nonetheless, there are some aspects of those issues that we lump together as 'insight' that do belong to the mentally ill person them self. People may be aware that they are mentally unwell, and yet they may not be able to identify those parts of their experience and behaviour that are attributable to illness, and which are not. They may understand that their elated mood is abnormal, and yet have no understanding of the effect that their behaviour is having on those around them. There are some other, more specific, psychopathological concepts that have greater utility than insight because they convey something more meaningful. For example, it is useful to think of people with autistic spectrum disorder as lacking a theory of mind, which is to say they cannot put themselves in other people's shoes in order to understand their thinking. They are constantly puzzled by reactions to their socially awkward behaviour. Stating that they lack insight conveys virtually no information, and is in any case untrue, because most people with autistic developmental problems are painfully aware that there is something different about them. Understanding their lack of a theory of mind allows an appreciation of their subjective experience of life. It also has some predictive value.

From time to time one comes across well-educated patients who affect a counterculture lifestyle. They can be frustrating to treat because they tend to sabotage attempts to stabilise their mental state. They commonly have achievable ambitions relating to the creative arts, which are thwarted by a chaotic pattern of illness, admission and remission. To a middle-aged psychiatrist, the chaos in these people's lives is frustrating because it appears to be avoidable. It often seems to be driven by childish and inconsequential decision making over serious matters such as medication, drug misuse and antisocial behaviour. One such patient of ours who suffered from bipolar affective disorder once said 'The manic episodes are your problem and the depressions are my problem.' He was only prepared to take responsibility for avoiding depression. His preferred method of achieving this was to take measures to push himself back into mania, with an inevitable pattern of readmissions as a consequence.

It seems to us that some of the sterile discussion as to whether the use of duress is justified by lack of insight would be more fruitfully reframed as a discussion over the extent to which people are prepared to take responsibility for improving their own mental health. This has to be approached with care, as there is a risk of blaming people for being ill, which is never appropriate, and of exacerbating depressive self-reproach over failure to recover by an act of will. However, many people who have continuous delusional beliefs (and therefore by definition 'lack insight') are prepared to take responsibility for their health. Their attitude to their beliefs is less important than their attitude towards their own well being.

Worried parents of adults with serious mental illness sometimes want the mental health services to use compulsion in order to control or eliminate delinquent behaviour, such as heavy cannabis use, that is volitional and difficult to influence. Service user groups tend to take the converse view. Many of them feel that mental health services do patients a disservice by allowing people to be absolved of responsibility for the direction of their lives. They feel that this leads to disempowerment. The dilemma of personal responsibility arises recurrently in clinical situations. Responsibility for one's actions is a key component of freedom. The dilemma is that neither removing personal responsibility nor keeping it with the patient at all times is a viable position. The key example of this dilemma concerns mentally disordered offenders.

Mentally disordered offenders

The McNaughton case was an important milestone in the liberalisation of attitudes to the mentally ill. It had an international impact. In 1843, Daniel McNaughton killed

Edward Drummond, private secretary to the Prime Minister, Sir Robert Peel. He acted on long-standing delusional beliefs. A group of lawyers and doctors, who believed it was wrong to hang the offender under these circumstances, successfully argued that he was not responsible for his actions. The verdict in the trial was novel: 'not guilty of murder by reason of insanity'. McNaughton spent the rest of his days in an asylum. There was, however, alarm amongst the British establishment over the verdict. The case was seen as a kind of miscarriage of justice, because McNaughton understood the nature of his actions (they were carefully planned) and he knew that he was breaking the law. A group of judges were given the task of setting out the circumstances under which such a defence could be used, in order to limit them. These became the 'McNaughton rules'.

On the one side, some saw McNaughton as an ill man who needed care (albeit in a secure setting). On the other side he was seen as a criminal deserving punishment, because, no matter what he believed, he knew he was committing a crime and the nature of the penalty. This tension between diametrically opposed ways of understanding mentally disordered offenders persists to this day.

Some social factors are associated with an increased risk of developing mental illness. These include growing up in poverty, poor educational attainment, and a range of other types of childhood and adult disadvantage. They are most prevalent in deprived inner-city areas. Exactly the same social factors are associated with criminality. It is therefore entirely predictable that mental illness should be common amongst offenders. Whilst there certainly are people who offend because they are mentally ill, many mentally disordered offenders develop mental illness against the background of an established pattern of offending behaviour. Is either group more or less culpable for offences committed when actively mentally ill? No reasonable person would blame those who are exposed to social disadvantage for developing a mental illness. Is it reasonable to blame mentally well offenders for their behaviour if they have been exposed to the same disadvantages? If we absolve the latter, what is our attitude to that large group of people who are exposed to disadvantage but lead blameless lives?

It seems very difficult to resolve these questions by reference to first principles. In reality, both mental health services and the legal system can only make rational and just decisions on the basis of individual circumstances and the likely consequences of punishment or treatment. However, even this is difficult. Britain has a major problem with prison overcrowding. This problem has worsened as criminal justice policies have increasingly emphasised long sentences. Prison authorities frequently complain that many of their inmates suffer from mental health problems, and they claim that they are now housing people who in the past would have been residents in large mental hospitals. This claim has been influential, although it does not correspond with the evidence (Leff *et al.*, 2000).

In the UK there is a long-standing policy that offenders who are mentally ill should be diverted away from penal custody and towards mental health services. Nearly all major cities have a criminal justice liaison scheme, staffed by mental health professionals. They are involved in helping the police and the courts by assessing offenders who appear to be mentally ill, arranging treatment and giving evidence where this is appropriate. They were initially named court diversion schemes, but their role has developed because in practice only a small minority of their clientele could be appropriately diverted to inpatient treatment. The modern role of forensic psychiatric services is focussed on the treatment of convicted prisoners, who are frequently transferred to NHS regional secure units.

These are welcome developments, but there is a continuing lack of agreement as to the criteria for treatment in place of punishment. There is no controversy over people who commit crimes as a direct consequence of the symptoms of psychosis, for example, acting under the influence of command hallucinations. There is far more difficulty when the relationship between offending and illness is more complicated. For example, some young men with schizophrenia are addicted to drugs. They recurrently commit robberies to fund their habit. There is a relationship between their addiction and their illness, but it is not one of simple causation. There is also a relationship between their illness and their offences, if only because being mentally unwell when you commit an offence makes it more likely that you will get caught. Treating the illness may have no influence on the addiction or offending. Absolving them of responsibility for offending can make it more difficult to persuade them to change their lifestyle. Punishing them by means of a custodial sentence rarely improves the situation.

We offer no solutions to these continuing dilemmas over personal responsibility, because there are none. This means that fixed rules are inappropriate, and that all such situations require careful thought before deciding what position is appropriate to adopt.

Is holistic care necessarily a good thing?

We have already explored the fact that there are many circumstances where it is important to attend to patients' general well being in order to help them overcome the effects of serious mental illness. Mental health services often need to assist people with housing problems, employment, education, physical health and so on. There is a down side in terms of dependency and stigma, but this is offset by greater benefits and progress towards the goal of recovery. However, there is a persistent demand that medicine in general and psychiatry in particular should become more holistic and less reductionist. Prince Charles, for example, made this the theme of his inaugural speech when he became Patron of the Royal College of Psychiatrists in the 1980s, and there has been a crescendo in this refrain from a variety of sources in the years that have followed. We strongly sympathise with criticism of an overemphasis on reductionism as a way of understanding people's problems. 'Holistic care', however, is a problematic model, not least because it embraces complementary therapies and attention to spirituality within treatment.

Complementary therapies are championed by some mental health professionals and are valued by some patients. The conventional medical view is that they are distinguished from orthodox therapies by the fact that they are based on unverifiable theories and by a lack of objective evidence that they work. If a central component of the legitimate role of psychiatry is the practical application of scientific knowledge, then involvement with complementary therapies can be seen as a betrayal of our professional obligations. Complementary therapies cost money and it can be argued that using them diverts resources from proper treatments. Some complementary medicines, such as Chinese herbal preparations, can be potent and therefore dangerous. Some such medicines have been found to contain toxins such as lead (Ernst, 2002). Invoking imaginary forces leads patients away from more tangible factors that can actually be changed in order to help them.

Set against this are some cogent counter-arguments. The theoretical basis for some orthodox treatments is hard to verify, and our theories often turn out to be wrong. There is little convincing evidence for many aspects of conventional treatment. Some complementary therapies have eventually been absorbed into the mainstream. Should we ignore the fact that some patients find complementary therapies helpful after they have found conventional approaches troublesome or ineffective? Should we regard psychoanalysis as a complementary or orthodox therapy?

It is, we think, impossible for mainstream psychiatry to embrace complementary therapies, but it is reasonable to adopt a position of skeptical tolerance. Blanket rejection and intolerance of complementary treatment in all its forms may be scientifically justifiable, but unavoidably creates an impression of inflexibility, and even bigotry, that is not compatible with a positive therapeutic stance.

Until recently, religion has been far less conspicuous in British life than is the case in most parts of the USA. However, the Zeitgeist has changed, and religious faith is playing an increasingly assertive role in public life. Against this general backdrop, there is mounting pressure within British psychiatry to attend to spiritual matters as part of treatment. 'Spirituality' is presented as an overarching concern that links all religions. The assertion is that there are important aspects of people's internal experience that are transcendent, and that warrant attention alongside more tangible domains. The suggestion that this might be divisive or sectarian is dismissed. Even atheists are said to have a spiritual life (though atheists tend to see this as nonsensical and a refusal to accept their rejection of religion).

It is important for psychiatrists to understand their patients' religious beliefs and practices, and the impact of these on their experience of mental illness. However, intervening at a spiritual level is, we believe, a serious breach of professional boundaries that can have adverse consequences for patients, even where they share the same religion as the clinician. Spiritual intervention is unequivocally the role of priests and religious elders, not doctors. We strongly believe that this aspect of 'holistic care' has to be resisted.

Main points in this chapter

1. Whilst issues concerning models of care may appear intangible and theoretical, they have an influence on day-to-day practice that is important.
2. Psychiatry characteristically moves between two models of care, each of which has strengths and weaknesses. It is helpful to maintain an awareness of which model you are applying.
3. 'Mental capacity' is an important and evolving concept that has to be understood, as it is likely to become increasingly important in the future.

4. The clinical constructs of mental capacity and personal responsibility contain ambiguities, which in turn create a range of practical dilemmas. Nonetheless, they probably have greater utility than the construct of 'insight'.

5. Comprehensive care and holistic care are different. The latter may not be an appropriate position for psychiatrists, as it leads away from the rational and the demonstrable and towards breaches of professional boundaries.

Part III - Problems in treatment

This section is concerned with the commonly occurring practical problems of treatment. These differ in type as treatment progresses. They can be broken down into difficulties in engagement, failure to agree to or to adhere to treatment plans, failure to get better, complications that impede progress, the management of problematic types of risk, and helping people to stay well in the long term. These problems are not necessarily due to factors belonging to the patient. Factors belonging to the clinician, contextual difficulties, and poor therapeutic relationships can all create significant impediments to recovery.

11 Engagement

The way that lives are led has a profound effect on physical and mental health. Personal well being depends on the things that people do each day. Unfortunately, no matter how healthy a lifestyle might be, everyone eventually develops illnesses and diseases that affect the ability to function. Technical treatments, such as medication, can control illness, but the existence of a technical treatment is not sufficient to return people to good health. Throughout medicine, and especially in psychiatry, patients have to participate in or co-operate with interventions if they are to be successful. They have to modify the things that they do every day in order to get better. Recovery is always an active process on the part of the patient.

Helping people to do the things that are necessary to recover is the core business of mental health care. It depends on the clinician's ability to form plans with patients, which involves continuing negotiation and discussion. This in turn is based on an important process that underlies all therapeutic progress. Treatment cannot progress unless the patient has engaged with the clinician.

Engagement is a first step and a continuing issue in treatment. It is a prerequisite to the formation of therapeutic relationships. Clinician and patient are both active agents in engagement. In clinical practice, *engagement* refers to the process by which clinician and patient start to do business with each other. Metaphorically they engage as cogs in a machine engage. Action on one side leads to a reciprocal movement on the other side. The process of engagement can be straightforward. You may be recommended to a patient by his general practitioner, and the patient may arrive with an expectation that you are likely to be helpful to him. During an initial interview, the patient comes to feel that you have understood him, and that you have proposed a treatment plan that is plausible and acceptable. Engagement has occurred effortlessly. The patient follows the plan that you have worked out together. However, the fact that an interview is cordial does not necessarily mean that engagement has occurred. Many patients retain a high level of skepticism or anxiety about psychiatric treatment without this being immediately evident.

The test of successful engagement is whether anything happens as a consequence of the interview. This may be a change in the way the patient thinks about their situation, or it may involve them doing something. Some patients are ostensibly happy with an initial interview, but return having failed to follow advice and with no change in their understanding of their problem. Nothing has happened as a consequence of the interview and engagement has not occurred.

Engagement can fail for a wide variety of reasons. The severity of the illness may make it impossible for the patient to engage at first. More frequently failure of engagement is related to factors concerning the two personalities and the interaction between them. Some patients with good 'insight' (i.e. a good understanding that they are mentally unwell) are difficult to engage because, like Diogenes, they just want to be left alone. Others with little 'insight' (i.e. a poor understanding of the nature of their problem) readily engage because they want help and because they trust health professionals. Some patients assiduously keep appointments over long periods of time and accumulate a good deal of face-to-face contact with clinicians without ever actually engaging with them. Some patients are forced unwillingly into a relationship with mental health services through the use of legal compulsion. Fortunately, most of these patients eventually start to engage with clinicians in the course of a relationship that commences under duress. Engaging patients who are initially reluctant is an essential skill for anyone involved in the treatment of serious mental illness.

Whilst engagement is necessary to allow a positive therapeutic relationship to flourish, engagement is not intrinsically therapeutically helpful. There are some circumstances where close engagement can be counter-therapeutic. We described a special and exclusive relationship between a team member and a patient that ultimately had a counter-therapeutic effect in Chapter 6 (Box 6.1). The patient engaged well with the community mental health nurse, but in such a way that it was impossible for her to engage with other mental health professionals. It was inevitable that circumstances would eventually arise where there would be a change of personnel, and this led directly to disengagement, relapse and a major setback for the patient. Engagement can lead to a destructively dependent relationship that undermines the patient's ability to solve their own problems.

Some clinicians try to achieve engagement through a type of dishonesty. This can take the form of making promises that cannot be honoured ('I will never detain you in hospital'). Some professionals maintain their personal engagement with the patient by disassociating themselves from some part of treatment. For example, when the patient has to be detained, they refuse to get involved or maintain a stance that this part of treatment had nothing to do with them. The implication to the patient is that, if they had made the decisions, things might have been different. The professional effectively disowns the legitimate and necessary actions of colleagues. This can be very destructive, as it hinders rather than assists in the process of agreeing a total package of care with the patient and it makes engagement with other team members more difficult. We do not suggest that mental health professionals should support colleagues who make avoidable errors or act inappropriately. However, teams and patients have to share an understanding that packages of care are, for the most part, irreducible. The component parts are dependant upon each other in order to achieve a successful outcome.

Engagement can be lost. Patients sometimes disengage because they feel let down, or because their circumstances change, or as part of a repetitive cycle of engagement and disengagement. Some patients disengage because they have recovered and correctly feel they need no further help, so they stop turning up for appointments.

Engagement is affected by factors belonging to the patient (for example, their life situation and their attitude to mental health services), factors belonging to the clinician (mainly their personality and their clinical skills) and factors within the relationship between them (for example, the degree to which personal characteristics mesh so that they can achieve a good rapport). Most of the qualities that a professional can use to enhance engagement are generally important in therapeutic relationships. In reiterating them here, we should mention a point that we have stressed elsewhere. Problems in therapeutic relationships almost always have their origins early on.

1. *Authenticity.* Patients find it easier to engage if they feel that they are making human contact with the clinician. This does not justify or necessitate breaking the boundaries of professional behaviour. It does not necessarily imply a need to like the patient. Authenticity rests on honesty, straight talking, and a degree of warmth in the interaction. Politeness and respectfulness should, of course, be the habitual stance of all clinicians, no matter who the patient is or how unwell they might be. However, rudeness is not the only route to a lack of warmth and authenticity. It is easy for professionals to appear patronising without realising it. An aloof or disinterested stance will put anyone off.

2. *Being heard.* People need to have their say. They need some indication that they have been heard, even if the clinician disagrees with them. Clinicians do not have to have an immediate solution to every problem. It is more important that they are properly attentive, and take care to understand what they are told. This means exploring patients' concerns, whatever they may be. There is evidence that psychiatrists have particular problems in discussing patients' concerns when they relate to the content of psychotic beliefs (McCabe *et al.*, 2002). Psychiatrists are interested in the nature and severity of psychotic symptoms and how they affect the patient's behaviour. It is more difficult for them to discuss, for example, the patient's frustration that neighbours are continuing to come into their property at night and move things around and that no one believes that the interference is really happening. Mental health professionals sometimes believe that it is harmful to discuss delusional beliefs because it somehow reinforces them. This is not true. There is a natural tendency to slide away from bizarre or paranoid topics, but this leaves patients feeling that they have not been listened to. Worries that are based on psychotic beliefs are hard to resolve, not least because the clinician does not believe that these things are actually happening. However, they are often the patients' most pressing concern, and the reason that they are seeking help. Patients are more likely to engage if their concerns are discussed and acknowledged. Developing the skill of talking about the content of psychotic symptoms in a therapeutically constructive way is difficult, but it is important in order to get alongside the patient.

3. *Gaining credibility.* Where engagement is difficult, gaining credibility with the patient makes a difference. Conversely, loss of credibility is a common prelude to disengagement. Credibility is enhanced by making sure that the things you say will happen do indeed happen. We have noted elsewhere that telling a patient that you are going to admit him to hospital for a few days rest when you intend a lengthier admission is a betrayal of a fundamental professional duty of honesty. It also sets up an inevitable loss of credibility when the patient eventually realises that you have been less than truthful. The resulting distrust is difficult to overcome. Helping to resolve practical

problems, such as organising assistance with financial or housing problems, can persuade the patient that you are going to be helpful in other ways. This type of credibility is particularly helpful in engaging those who are routinely most difficult to engage, namely people who are living at the margins of society and who are suspicious of authority. Credibility can be established at any stage in treatment, including very late on (see Box 11.1).

Box 11.1 It is never too late to establish your credibility

Amanda was a thirty-five-year-old graduate who lived with her parents and worked in the family furniture business. She had developed bipolar affective disorder at the age of twenty-two, and suffered regular relapses of mania. She would be admitted for two to three weeks after an abrupt onset of disturbed behaviour. Once her mental state improved she would become very embarrassed over her disinhibition, and she usually suffered several months of depression thereafter.

Amanda disliked medication. She was tried on a variety of mood stabilisers, antidepressants and antipsychotics, but found none of them satisfactory. She would agree to only low or sub-threshold doses of medication. She rejected psychological work to allow her to manage her condition through the recognition of early warning signs and self-medication because this too involved medication. She accepted visits from a community mental health nurse, and would chat with her cheerfully enough when well. When depressed she was withdrawn and passively accepted medication administered by her mother. Her relationship with the team psychiatrist was difficult. She tried to keep interviews with him to a minimum. When they did meet she was sullen and uncommunicative, and the discussion centred on her unhappiness with the current medication.

Things changed as a consequence of a discussion with the nurse about her sense that life was passing her by, and that she had a diminishing chance of having a career or finding a partner. The nurse told her that she and the psychiatrist were also concerned about the pattern of illness that seemed to be preventing her from getting on with her life. Amanda reacted with incredulity, and said that it seemed to her that all the mental health services seemed interested in was subduing her through the use of drugs. The nurse suggested that, if this was what she believed, it might be illuminating for her to read her case notes.

After Amanda read her case notes, her relationship with the clinicians abruptly changed. She requested work to follow a self-management strategy, and her interviews with both the doctor and nurse became more constructive. The cycle of relapse was broken. She now admitted that she had never actually taken medication for any length of time, but that when it was necessary, the side effects were tolerable. The change, she said, was due to the attitudes displayed in the case notes. She had expected critical comments. Instead, they were objective, and it was clear that the professionals really had been concerned about the problems in her life all along. The team had suddenly gained credibility and for the first time, she engaged with them properly.

4. *Clarity.* You cannot expect patients to engage with you unless they understand your intentions. This means that interactions should usually end with a clear explanation of the overall plan (if you have formed one) and what you intend to do next. Transparency and clarity are important principles at all stages of every type of mental health intervention. There is nothing more likely to make a therapeutic relationship fail than confusion over the formulation of the problem and the treatment plan. During engagement, clarity helps patients to decide whether to trust you. It can relieve unspoken anxieties over what you might do.

5. *Anticipating problems.* If there are obvious factors that might make engagement difficult, such as a previous bad experience of psychiatric treatment or anxiety that children may be taken into care, it is usually best to acknowledge and discuss them at an early stage. It is not the case that you can give an absolute assurance that feared consequences will not occur. However, the process of identifying and talking through these fears can make it easier for patients to relax, which makes engagement more likely. Under many circumstances, involvement with services is actually the patients' best protection against feared outcomes, and people can only come to see this if it is openly discussed.

6. *Persistence.* If patients do not engage quickly, it is tempting to give up. This may be appropriate under some circumstances. When risks appear small, or treatment is contingent upon motivation (for example, psychotherapy or intervention for addiction), it can be seriously unhelpful to press help too hard. Untoward pressure to engage in treatment can make it less likely that the patient will engage at a later stage, when something has changed. On the other hand, in the treatment of severe mental illness it can be impossible for the patient to ever recover unless services take an assertive stance. This can mean a degree of persistence and a firm reluctance to take no for an answer.

7. *Willingness to apologise when things go wrong.* Apologies can be important in avoiding disengagement. A sincere apology over unexpected side effects, or a remark that has been taken the wrong way, is engaging, so long as it is unequivocal. An apology should include an explanation as to how things went wrong. This is different from an apology that is followed by an assertion that it was not really your fault anyway, or worse, that it was actually somebody else's fault. These half-apologies are alienating, as is obvious to anyone who has ever complained to a call centre about a loss of an essential utility.

Engagement involves the use of personal social skills to achieve a clinical objective. Everyone finds some types of people easier to engage with than others, and this is largely a reflection of how easily the two personalities mesh. It is not necessarily the case that people have to have a lot in common. For example, there is a wide variation amongst clinicians in their ability to understand and engage marginalised people with unusual (or deviant) lifestyles. Those clinicians who can do this with ease are often well-educated, middle-class people with relatively conventional lifestyles. The ability seems to be a reflection of personality characteristics. Sometimes these clinicians have greater difficulty in engaging patients with similar backgrounds to their own. In our experience, when deciding which team member should try to engage a patient, it is much more important to take into account these personal preferences than it is to worry too much about specific skills that the professional possesses. Engagement is the first priority because specific skills can only be deployed once the patient has engaged.

Team engagement

There are often discussions within CMHTs as to whether a particular patient has engaged 'with the team'. In reality, no one ever engages with a whole team. Discussion about failure to engage with the team arises because the patient is in contact with several team members and has not engaged with any of them. Patients engage with individual clinicians. No one could engage with something so intangible as a team. Patients who engage well with one clinician often engage easily with other team members. This is not the same as collective engagement. Once the patient has had a positive experience with one professional, the task of engagement is much easier next time.

The fact that engagement is a phenomenon that occurs between two people has a practical importance, because many mental health professionals work in large teams. One cannot deploy team members interchangeably and expect to maintain patients' engagement. Many Assertive Outreach Teams (AOTs) in the UK follow the model developed by Stein and Test (1980) in Madison, Wisconsin, known as Psychiatric Assertive Community Treatment (PACT). One of the principles of PACT is that all patients and treatment plans should be known to the whole team, so that there is consistency when the patient's key worker is not available. Some AOTs appear to have taken this to mean that individual therapeutic relationships are to be avoided. All team members visit all patients, and the patient may not know who is going to visit on a given day until they arrive. AOTs exist for patients who have difficulty in engaging constructively with mental health professionals. In our opinion, randomising staff can only make engagement more difficult. Even where there is no such randomisation, there is a limit to the number of professionals that a patient can engage with simultaneously. In our experience this is usually three or four. Even people who are keen to engage struggle to do so beyond this limit.

When a patient is in contact with several team members, the degree and quality of engagement with each of them varies. This is particularly true when working with people suffering from chronic active psychosis. Under these circumstances, the team member who tends to have the greatest problem in engaging the patient is generally the psychiatrist. The psychiatrist has the least face-to-face contact with the patient, and may be perceived as the primary agent in the least welcome aspects of treatment. Community nurses, on the other hand, are in frequent contact with the patient and tend to deliver the most acceptable aspects of treatment, such as the resolution of practical difficulties. There is a pitfall here. The clinicians can find themselves in a 'good cop, bad cop' position, a dysfunctional splitting of care into the acceptable and unacceptable. To avoid this, the psychiatrist has to continue to put effort into engaging the patient, rather than following the line of least resistance by leaving everything to the community nurse.

Some patients move through a cycle of engagement and disengagement determined by changes in their mental health, but team factors can also lead to disengagement. For example, lengthy periods of staff sickness can be highly problematic, especially where an alternative team member takes over on a temporary basis. The transient nature of the relationship can lead to delays in pursuing treatment plans ('this is something you can get on with once Brian is back'), with a resultant sense of inactivity and disillusionment that can lead to disengagement. Equally, the arrival of a new psychiatrist, with different ideas about medication and treatment plans, can be a breath of fresh air for a team, but it can derail treatment that is working well. Even if the patient does not completely disengage, he can remain very attached to the previous psychiatrist, making proper engagement difficult for the current psychiatrist ('Dr Owen told me not to stop these tablets unless he told me, and I had a lot of faith in Dr Owen'). This type of persistent attachment to obsolete advice can outlive the psychiatrist by several decades.

Difference

The existence of differences between clinicians and patients is not necessarily a barrier to engagement. As we have pointed out, some professionals have the greatest difficulty working with those patients who are most like themselves. Many aspects of the human experience tell us that rapport and close relationships can form between people who ostensibly have little in common. However, it would be foolish to deny that some types of difference can be a major obstruction to engagement. Lack of a common language is a good example. Even the use of an exemplary translation service can only allow a limited degree of rapport and engagement. In routine work, the difference that most commonly causes an obstruction to engagement is when clinician and patient belong to social groups that have major differences in power, and when the patient suffers discrimination and prejudice in everyday life.

In the UK, young men from families of Afro-Caribbean origin are more likely to be diagnosed as suffering from schizophrenia than the rest of the population. They are overrepresented amongst those detained under the Mental Health Act and amongst mentally disordered offenders. They are more likely to be dissatisfied with mental health services than other patients (Parkman *et al.*, 1997). There is controversy over the reasons for this, but one can say with some certainty that mental health services do not engage well with young black men. Young black men experience discrimination in their lives in a range of ways, and it is understandable that they approach mental health services with some apprehension. However, having worked in an ethnically diverse area for many years, we have to say that we have never found young black men any more suspicious or alienated than other young men. There is evidence to support our impression (Priebe *et al.*, 2005). The problem in engaging young black men may lie in interactions when they first come into contact with mental health services. Clinicians can be affected by prevalent social stereotypes, some of which suggest that young black men are suspicious, anti-authority and potentially violent. This may lead the clinician to expect problems, and apprehension of this sort is bound to be evident, rendering engagement more difficult. A professional who starts an interview with a belief that the patient is going to be difficult is unlikely to seem warm and relaxed. Clinicians have to recognise that differences between groups of people are superficial. People are fundamentally all the same. There are excellent reasons to behave in the same way towards everyone.

Differences in sexual orientation, religion, class and culture can cause similar problems. Gender difference causes a different type of difficulty. Sexism is by no means dead, and there is still a real power difference between men and women. Moreover, men and women have some powerful models of relationship which can influence interactions in a dysfunctional way. These are:

- mother/son
- father/daughter
- brother/sister
- potential lovers
- spouse

These models are familiar and comfortable for most people, though their presence in therapeutic relationships is rarely explicit or acknowledged outside of psychoanalysis, where they are subsumed into the concept of transference. During engagement there is a pitfall whereby one party or the other slips into a version of one of these models, which will tend to lead the other party to follow their cues. This reciprocal pattern invites a breach of boundaries, although in the more common scenario, interactions take on some features of these models without anything improper happening. This still causes real problems for patients, for example, for women who have suffered abuse at the hands of a partner, or for men who hold angry feelings towards maternal figures. Whilst problems of this general type can occur in same-sex relationships (for example, for men who hold anger to paternal figures), they have a particular potency across genders. It can be tempting to imagine that engagement can be facilitated by exploiting one of these templates. A kind of flirtatious banter or a parental stance may seem to ease the establishment of the relationship. However, it plants the seeds of problems later, when the patient (and sometimes the clinician) can become quite confused over the boundaries of the relationship. Although gender difference between clinician and patient is commonplace it deserves attention and a degree of sensitivity.

We have written elsewhere (Poole & Higgo, 2006) about overcoming problems of difference, but suffice to say that one of the ways to overcome them involves identifying and understanding them, and sharing the problem with the patient (who is likely to be just as aware of the problem as you are).

Respect and dignity

There is a basic human need for respect and dignity. The service user movement has been very consistent in telling us that a loss of self-respect and dignity is one of the worst aspects of suffering from a mental illness. There is unanimity amongst policy makers, professionals and service users that patients' need for respect and dignity should be attended to at all times. However, we are a long way from consistently achieving this.

Indeed, there is an equally large problem in hospital medicine in general, where patients are commonly treated in ways that are an affront to personal dignity.

For professionals, the key difficulty seems to be the legitimate need to say and do things that patients may find difficult. Because we do and say things that are outside of the repertoire of normal social behaviour, some professionals deal with the discomfort of the situation by resorting to one of two equally poor solutions. The first is to infantilise patients, by behaving as if they are dim-witted or naughty children. The second is to avoid difficult topics altogether, for example, by failing to tell patients that you intend to detain them or by failing to tell them that you believe that they suffer from schizophrenia. Neither stance is compatible with dignity and respect, and there are far reaching consequences in the therapeutic relationship. It is perfectly possible to challenge people and to say difficult things to them whilst behaving respectfully towards them. It does not involve a complex technique. It requires a degree of frankness which the majority of patients welcome. What is difficult is coping with one's own discomfort. This diminishes with practice. It is a nettle that has to be grasped by all mental health professionals.

Expectations regarding conduct only work if they are reciprocal. It is very difficult to behave respectfully towards someone if they are being threatening or offensive towards you, in other words, if they fail to observe your need for dignity and respect too. Polite and respectful behaviour will nearly always be reciprocated, even by people who are suffering from severe psychosis. When people are very ill and behaving in a way that you find unacceptable, calmly insisting that the conversation can only continue if they are civil often leads to an immediate change in their behaviour. This does not imply an expectation that the patient should be deferential. An expectation of civility is an intrinsic component of mutual respect between autonomous human beings. An acceptance of unpleasant behaviour is infantilising, and encourages further regression. As the earliest contact between mental health professionals and patients can occur when the patient is very ill, the expectation of civility on both sides is relevant to the task of engaging people who are acutely disturbed.

Of course, some people really cannot control their behaviour, particularly people who are manic. Unlike inpatient mental health nurses, psychiatrists can keep interactions short under these circumstances. The principle, however, is to continue to insist that the patient should observe the normal rules of conduct. Observing these rules oneself in the face of difficult behaviour tends to hasten a return to normal standards of social interaction, even before the patient has fully recovered.

In recent years there has been a growth in zero-tolerance policies amongst mental health services. It is impossible to disagree with the principle that mental health professionals should not have to endure abuse, intimidation or violence in the course of their work. However, zero-tolerance policies dictate that patients should be treated as if entirely responsible for their actions at all times, and that mental illness is irrelevant to their conduct. The police are involved at the same threshold as would apply to the actions of someone who is mentally well. Zero-tolerance policies can have no exceptions by definition. This position is unsustainable. It is bound to take you to a place where you do not want to go. Few conscientious mental health professionals could feel comfortable in asking the police to charge a very ill patient who has made a minor assault on them as a direct consequence of psychosis. The stance is also incompatible with the legal concept of *mens rea* (the ability to form a culpable intention to break the law). It is an affront to natural justice, and, if pursued to its logical conclusion, results in ill people being punished by the service that is supposed to care for them. We accept that people should be held responsible for their actions unless there are strong grounds to believe otherwise, and this is as true for people with mental illness as anybody else. We fully accept that managers of mental health services must protect their staff. We do suggest that the application of policies on acceptable behaviour always demands a degree of judgement and, sometimes, tolerance.

In the fullness of time, very ill patients get better, and they often apologise for their behaviour. There is a reflex urge to respond to the effect that no apology is necessary, because they were ill at the time. Although well meaning, this is an error. Accepting the apology is polite and marks a clear restoration of normal rules of social interaction. Dismissal of the apology is a covert refusal to acknowledge the other person's right to own their behaviour, even when it is influenced by factors beyond their control.

We are aware that there is a degree of contradiction in the above. We are suggesting that an insistence on mutually respectful and civil behaviour is an essential component of appropriate therapeutic relationships, but that sometimes one has to tolerate unacceptable behaviour. We cannot resolve this paradox, but we observe that the critical and problematic judgement is in deciding where the boundary between the two lies.

Main points in this chapter

1. Engagement means that something happens as a consequence of therapeutic interviews, even if it is only a change in the way that patients understand their situations.
2. Engagement is necessary for therapeutic progress to occur, but it is not sufficient in itself. Some ways of engaging patients can be anti-therapeutic and counterproductive.
3. Engagement can be lost, and some patients see mental health professionals for long periods of time without ever engaging with them.
4. The factors that facilitate engagement are similar to those that promote positive therapeutic relationships in general.
5. Patients engage with individual professionals, not whole teams. There is a limit to the number of people someone can engage with simultaneously.
6. Difference and differential power can impede engagement, but there are steps that individual clinicians can take to overcome this.
7. Respect for patients, and their personal dignity, is supported by polite frankness and an expectation of reciprocal standards of conduct.

12 Compliance and concordance

Traditionally, adherence to medical advice has been conceptualised as *compliance*. This is now seriously out of fashion. Indeed, an otherwise sympathetic academic reviewer of our proposal for this book was appalled that we intended to use the term 'compliance' at all. There are a number of good reasons to reject compliance as a desirable objective. Compliance implies a passive submission to the doctor's will. It is based on the assumption that medical advice is necessarily good advice, which is not always the case (in the fullness of time, accepted medical wisdom can prove to be wrong, for example, the use of bed rest for low back pain, or prefrontal leucotomy for schizophrenia). Even when advice is sound, individual circumstances can make it inappropriate or impossible to implement. In any case, the gap between the level of education and information of doctors and patients has narrowed. The authoritarian, all-knowing doctor directing the deferentially compliant patient was never a good model, and it is untenable in the present day.

Much of the modern literature concerning adherence to treatment plans suggests that the concept of compliance should be replaced by *concordance*. Concordance means that the clinician and patient agree on a treatment plan and adhere to it. When the patient fails to take prescribed medication, the problem can be understood in a number of different ways, which prominently includes failure to achieve true agreement between psychiatrist and patient over the treatment plan in the first place. The advantage of this way of thinking is that it allows the clinician to search for strategies that will move the situation forward. The process of finding an effective plan that can be willingly followed is a therapeutic and co-operative enterprise that engages patients and professionals as partners. Understanding the problem as non-compliance, on the other hand, locates the problem entirely within the patient, who is simply not doing as they are told. This invites the doctor to try to resolve the situation by exerting authority, an approach that rarely works.

Working towards concordance is an important theme in psychiatric treatment. However, whilst concordance is an objective in all cases, it is not invariably achieved. Some patients reluctantly comply with treatment as one stage along the path to concordance. Some therapeutic relationships never move beyond this point. When patients comply with treatment because of duress or deference, it is misleading to suppose that this is a form of concordance. Compliance is less robust than concordance because agreements are mature arrangements that can be modified, whereas obedience is an infantilising phenomenon that invites rebellion. In clinical practice it is important to recognise the difference between compliance and concordance. From time to time one hears mental health professionals make comments such as 'The patient is non-concordant'. This is a semantic nonsense. What is meant is that the patient is non-compliant. The professional has changed the words, but they have failed to understand or to alter their thinking. As is usually the case, the use of a euphemism clouds the issue.

Much of this chapter concerns medication. Medication is often an essential component of treatment, necessary but not sufficient to achieve recovery. Few patients with recurrent or chronic psychosis can remain well without sometimes using medication. However, in focussing on medication, we do not seek to reify it. There is much more to successful treatment than medication, and many of the considerations explored here apply equally to concordance with psychological and social interventions.

Why don't patients do as they are told?

> Look, this really is very simple. You suffer from a mental illness that is, in its nature, recurrent. When you are ill you go through absolute torment. Your family is very distressed every time you relapse. The medication works perfectly well for you. It is true that you have some side effects, but they are trivial in the face of the destruction that repeated admissions to hospital cause in your life. You don't deny that you have this illness, and you accept that the medication works, but over and again you stop taking your tablets without telling anyone, on some spurious rationale. Sure as night follows day, within a few weeks you are severely unwell, and then I have to admit you to hospital and pick up the pieces. Why on earth won't you just do as you are told?

Perhaps there are psychiatrists who never think like this, but we doubt it. Sometimes a clear exposition of the situation as you see it can be quite helpful, because frankness and honesty are always sound principles. However, this is only likely to work if the psychiatrist has a good understanding of the reasons why the patient stops medication. Without this, the relationship with the patient goes seriously wrong when this type of thinking takes over. The sentiment captured by the sentence 'Why on earth don't you just do as you are told?' is frustration and irritation. These feelings are underpinned by 'I have to pick up the pieces'. The patient's failure to take the tablets frustrates the psychiatrist because he has come to see relapses as a problem to him, not to the patient and his family. The patient is well and rational when he chooses to discontinue medication, so the psychiatrist tends to feel that the patient is being wilfully defiant and making life difficult. Compliance becomes a power struggle. This makes things worse, because many patients then conceal their non-compliance. If there was no power struggle, this would not be necessary. It is probably inevitable that some therapeutic relationships will travel down this dead end sometimes, but we can say from bitter experience, it is entirely fruitless. After a few years trapped with the patient in this position, you end up feeling bad tempered and ineffectual, which is exactly what you are for this particular patient. To avoid this, it is useful to think about adherence to treatment in a different way.

One of the most important things that the clinician has to recognise is that it is intrinsically difficult to accept that your sanity depends on taking medication, especially when you are symptom free. This is in part related to the stigma associated with mental illness. One of us was recently chatting to the cashier at a local petrol station, a young man who he sees quite regularly as an anonymous customer. The cashier mentioned that he had some health problems. 'In fact,' he said 'I'm a diagnosed schizophrenic, but don't worry, I'm perfectly safe'. It is hardly surprising that it is difficult to accept that you suffer from schizophrenia continuously when you know that strangers will automatically, but erroneously, assume that you are therefore dangerous. Denial of the implications of the diagnosis is entirely understandable.

Stigma is not necessarily the most important barrier to accepting a diagnosis of severe mental illness. There is a more profound emotional difficulty in accepting that it could all come back if you stop taking medication. For many people the psychological need to feel whole again demands that they should prove to themselves and the world that they can be well without medication. The fact of taking medication is a daily reminder that they are in some way not restored and it drags them back into the illness experience with all its resonances of being less than other people.

Sometimes, in an effort to get people suffering from schizophrenia to accept depot antipsychotic injections, a parallel is drawn with diabetes. Just like the person with diabetes, it is said, you need to take the injections to correct a problem with your body's chemistry. If you do this, you can get on with your life like anybody else. There is nothing fundamentally flawed in the simile, but what it overlooks is the fact that all diabetologists recognise the problem of treating young people who will not adhere to their insulin regime. They fail to adhere to treatment plans for exactly the same reasons as young people suffering from schizophrenia. They want to be 'normal' and find it extremely difficult to accept that they have a long-term health problem when they feel perfectly well.

It is easier to work with people who are struggling with the effect on their self-perception in this way if you understand that the adjustment involved is painful, and that it takes time to overcome it. Battering people with the facts tends to deepen their denial, whereas trying to work with the emotional distress that underlies it tends to be more fruitful.

Adjustment to the diagnosis of psychotic illness does not just affect the patient. Families have to deal with it too, and this can have an impact on adherence to treatment plans. Sometimes this is quite apparent, sometimes less so. It is common for families to identify genuine psychological factors and stresses that have played a part in the person becoming unwell. Many come to the understandable and logical conclusion that psychotherapy might correct the underlying cause of the illness. Psychotherapy has a significant role in helping people with serious mental illness, but it rarely obviates the need for medication when people are suffering from schizophrenia or bipolar affective disorder. Families can come to see these treatment modalities as polar opposites, which can then create a dilemma for the patient who has to choose between the opinion of the professionals and the opinion of the family. Sometimes family resistance to treatment plans is more complex and less logical, and this can make it harder to identify. One of the advantages of working with patients in their own homes and amongst the people who are important to them is that these problems can be more easily tackled.

There is a wide variety of factors that can make it difficult for people to adhere to treatment plans, and they can only be overcome if they are understood. The reasons for resisting treatment are not trivial, and getting alongside patients means searching together for ways around problems.

'Non-compliance is not an option'

In 1998, Paul Boateng, at that time the British government minister with responsibility for mental health, made a statement that set out the underlying ethos of UK government policy on mental health. He said:

> We must make sure that we don't allow a culture of non-compliance with medication and therapy which precipitates breakdown. What we can say [to patients] is that if you are to remain in the community at large you must complete your medication and therapy. If you don't then the law gives clinicians the power to bring you back to a place of greater safety for yourself and the wider community. (Anon., 1998)

This statement caused outrage amongst the whole mental health community, because it was clearly based on prejudiced attitudes and factual errors. One of the factual errors was the existence of a 'culture of non-compliance'. It is true that a significant proportion of hospital admissions are associated with discontinuation of medication. It is flawed logic to conclude from this that people with mental illness are particularly prone to 'poor compliance'. In fact, rates of treatment adherence for people with schizophrenia and depression are similar to the rates for people suffering from chronic physical illness (Cramer & Rosenheck, 1998). The general population is very poor at adhering to instructions regarding medication. A large proportion of all prescriptions in general practice are not taken as directed and one study showed that 14.5% of prescriptions were not even collected from the pharmacist (Beardon *et al.*, 1993). A high proportion of all dispensed medication sits in bathroom cabinets until it is thrown away, several years after its use-by date. On the other hand, about 58% of people prescribed antipsychotics and 65% people prescribed antidepressants take their medication as directed (Cramer & Rosenheck, 1998). People with mental illness are much the same as everyone else when it comes to following treatment plans.

Adhering to treatment plans is meaningless unless they offer a route back to good health and the life that the person wants. People with mental illness have to be recognised as the individuals with the biggest stake in their own well being and therefore autonomous partners in the project. To characterise them as feckless and reckless in their attitude to treatment, so that they have to be threatened into compliance, is a counsel of despair. It seldom works in the long run, and it is very difficult to move from threats to partnership. There is a tiny minority of people with mental illness who are either severely ill, or who are indeed feckless and reckless, so that they cannot safely take responsibility for their own well being. They loom large in the awareness of professionals, because they cause us a lot of concern, and their treatment takes up a disproportionate amount of our time. However, this is not the generality, and even those who fall into a high-risk, treatment-avoiding group do change with time and skilful management. The process of negotiation over the nature of the problem and the most appropriate way of solving it drives the movement from compliance to concordance. This is the central dynamic in the development of a constructive therapeutic relationship with people suffering from severe mental illness.

Why do patients adhere to treatment plans?

Psychotropic medications are problematic. They are an important and necessary part of treatment. However, there are marked limitations to their effectiveness, and they can have persistent and unpleasant side effects. Although the introduction of SSRIs and 'atypical' antipsychotic drugs was said to herald an era of more tolerable psychotropic medications, in the fullness of time, disappointment has set in. The newer medications have different side effects to the older ones, and the existence of a wider range of drugs has been helpful in some ways (though it has also tended to encourage the frequent medication changes which we believe to be counter-productive). The fact that, for example, more than 50% of people with schizophrenia take medication as prescribed is arresting in the light of the barriers to accepting that it is necessary and the range of side effects that most patients experience. The evidence on the effectiveness of interventions to improve treatment adherence in severe mental illness is equivocal, but there are some clear messages about the factors associated with adherence.

Although side effects and 'insight' are relevant to adherence to treatment plans, neither appears to be the critical factor. It is true that people who have a good understanding of their illness and those who suffer fewer side effects seem to find treatment easier to accept. However, many patients with little or no side effects do not take their medication, and many patients with quite severe side effects do. Furthermore, many patients with poor 'insight' adhere to treatment plans, and some patients with a good understanding do not (Day *et al.*, 2005).

Overall, younger people and those who are socially marginalised are less likely to stick to plans. Older people and those who are socially integrated are more likely to do so. However, the most important factor appears to be the quality of the relationship with the treating clinician. Attitudes to psychiatric treatment matter, but these are formed by the experience of being treated by individual professionals. This is evident in clinical practice. Building a good relationship with a 'difficult' patient can transform the overall situation. The process of getting alongside people does seem to make a real difference to their ability to own and eventually manage their own illness. The findings with regard to age and social integration may be due to differences in general attitudes to authority and health professionals, which can make the process easier or more difficult. Of course, a part of engagement involves taking the patient's views and concerns seriously. There is nothing mystical about good therapeutic relationships. Anyone would be likely to follow a plan that they understand and have played a part in forming, especially if they trust the clinician and know that, if treatment causes them problems, this will be dealt with (Day *et al.*, 2005).

Side effects

Trying to minimise side effects is an important objective in itself, and taking side effects seriously is part of the clinician's task in achieving concordance. Psychiatrists and patients can have rather different ideas about side effects. With regard to antipsychotics, for example, psychiatrists worry most about extrapyramidal side effects (especially akathisia), changes to cardiac conduction and metabolic problems such as diabetes. Patients are very bothered by feeling drugged, by weight gain and by sexual side effects. It is not that one set of priorities is more important than the other. However, there is a danger that the patient's priorities are neglected, and this is an understandable route to unilateral decisions to discontinue medication.

The fundamental principle in avoiding sudden discontinuation of treatment is to explain to patients what effects they can expect from the medication, including time scale. This has been recognised for decades, but this is still commonly neglected by doctors in all branches of medicine. It may be that time pressures deter practitioners from fully explaining drug effects, but if so, it is a false time economy, because it takes longer to persuade patients to resume a drug they have stopped (or to take a different one). It is possible that doctors avoid discussing side effects because they fear that patients will be more likely to notice them if they are forewarned, or that they will be put off from taking the medication in the first place if they are well informed of likely side effects. It is hard to know if such fears are justified, but needless to say, it is perfectly evident that warning people is the superior strategy, because it is associated with a lower rate of discontinuation.

Drugs come in packages that contain patient information leaflets. These are not a substitute for explaining things to the patient. The leaflets are overinclusive and defensive, and it is not surprising that people sometimes read them and decide that the risks of the medication are too enormous to be tolerated. The therapeutic effects and side effects of medication are rarely synchronous, and without information this can persuade people that the side effects are prominent whilst the therapeutic effects are minimal or non-existent. For example, SSRI antidepressants tend to cause significant nausea in the first few days of treatment, but the therapeutic benefit takes longer to appear. No one can tolerate nausea indefinitely, but most people can put up with it for a few days until it passes in the expectation of a likely benefit later on.

Effects that are welcomed early in treatment can become problematic in a later phase. For example, the sedative effects of antipsychotic medication are often perceived as a welcome calming effect when people are suffering from acute psychosis and are feeling very anxious. This can turn into an unpleasant drugged feeling when acute symptoms have subsided. Clinicians should continue to actively enquire about side effects throughout treatment, no matter how well tolerated a medication has been initially. It is always best to ask people 'What medication are you taking?' and 'What dose?' because if they are taking it irregularly or at a lower than prescribed dose they will tell you, whereas if you ask 'Are you taking the medication?' they will equally honestly say that they are. Similarly, it is always best to ask 'Have you noticed anything that might be a side effect?' because it opens up a dialogue that allows problems to be discussed before they have passed the threshold of unacceptability.

In our experience, some approaches work much better than others in trying to minimise side effects. The second worst strategy is serial changes of drug, because once you have changed the medication twice because of side effects it is extremely rare for any of the next half a dozen drugs to prove any more satisfactory. When this happens, the patient quite frequently ends up deciding that, in the light of experience, the first drug was not too bad, and all that has happened is that improvement has been delayed by weeks or months. The absolute worst strategy is to change to the newest drug on the market, which almost invariably will have been recently promoted by the pharmaceutical company as being better tolerated than older drugs. Having seen many new drugs launched, it is evident that such claims are highly likely to prove over-optimistic. By routinely offering a drug that is something of an unknown quantity, you are taking a gamble, whereas if you change to a drug that you are very familiar with, you are able to give the patient a much more accurate account of likely effects.

We find the following principles helpful in minimising side effects:

- *Is the problem really due to the drug?* This is particularly important where the problem is known to be a potential side effect, but can have other causes. For example, daytime somnolence is a common side effect of higher doses of all antipsychotics. However, when people complain of sleeping all day, it is often because the structure of their life has collapsed, and they are sitting up into the early hours watching television, with the inevitable consequence that they have to catch up on sleep in the daytime. They are then wide awake at a normal bedtime and a vicious cycle commences (the same problem can arise with teenage children). This problem cannot be resolved by altering the drug regime, though occasionally a short course of night sedation is useful in re-establishing a normal sleep cycle. On the other hand, some depressed patients taking tricyclic antidepressants complain that they sleep for more than twelve hours a day, but on closer enquiry it emerges that they are in bed but awake, unable to face the world. This may mean that treatment is not working, but it does not mean that they are oversedated.

- *How much is it bothering the patient?* Sometimes patients are happy to tolerate a side effect if they know that it is due to the drug and that it is reversible. The fact that they mention a side effect does not necessarily mean that they want you to do anything about it. For example, one of the more troublesome side effects of clozapine is drooling. Some patients are very bothered by this, but others who only drool in their sleep feel that the side effect is a bearable penalty in the face of the benefit of the superior symptom relief that clozapine achieves. This must be the patient's decision. It is one thing to work with patients to assess the cost–benefit balance of a treatment. It is quite another thing to try to persuade them that a side effect that is distressing them is not really a problem at all.

- *Is this a bizarre or implausible side effect?* You have to be very careful about peculiar side effects, because sometimes the patient is right. For example, in the early days of the use of sodium valproate as a mood stabiliser, one of our patients complained that it had made her hair go curly. This seemed completely implausible until the literature was checked and it was found to be a recognised side effect. Clear and convincing accounts of side effects that are not recognised in the literature nearly always mean that the patient has noticed something that science has overlooked. Patients complained of withdrawal symptoms on stopping antidepressants long before this was generally recognised by psychiatrists as a real and common problem. However, sometimes patients who complain of strange side effects are communicating something else. Some patients with psychosis come to attribute psychotic symptoms to the medication. Some patients complain of peculiar side effects of medication because they do not trust the prescriber and are making a *post hoc* rationalisation of a wish to stop treatment.

- *What is the overall burden of side effects?* Given that all drugs have side effects, one prominent side effect may be easier to manage than a number of less severe side effects, in which case a change of drug may make things worse, not better.
- *Can the problem be resolved or improved by a reduction in dosage?* Prescribers seem to find it relatively easy to increase doses or add drugs, but are much more anxious about reducing drugs or stopping them altogether. This concern is not altogether without foundation, but provided dosage reductions are made slowly, sudden relapses are uncommon because exact doses of psychotropic agents are rarely critical to effectiveness. Even quite modest dosage reductions can make the difference between intolerable and bearable side effects.
- *Can dosage schedules be altered so that side effects are intermittent rather than continuous?* Licensing authorities continue to insist that pharmaceutical companies recommend dosage schedules that lead to pharmacokinetic stability (i.e. the steadiest possible blood level over twenty-four hours). Some drugs, notably antidepressants, only seem to work if this stability is achieved. However, this is not necessary for therapeutic benefit with some other drug treatments. For most patients, antipsychotic medication can be taken once a day without a loss of benefit, irrespective of the drug's pharmacokinetics. A once-a-day regime, particularly at bedtime, can minimise daytime side effects. This is not a panacea. The regime can cause morning drowsiness in some people.
- *Can the side effect be managed non-pharmacologically?* Weight gain is a problem with many psychotropic medications, and can be a severe problem for patients taking some antipsychotics, e.g. clozapine and olanzapine. Sometimes weight gain is so rapid and so severe that there is no alternative but to change medications, but sometimes it can be tackled through specific work on lifestyle, diet and exercise.
- *Is adding a drug to control the side effect likely to improve things?* Antimuscarinic agents have a well-established role in controlling extra pyramidal side effects, and small doses of a beta-blocker sometimes eliminate akathisia. However, antimuscarinic agents can worsen concentration or short-term memory, especially in older people, and beta-blockers can be lethal for people with asthma. If a drug is added, how long do you intend to continue it? If you are unclear about this, it is likely to be prescribed in perpetuity and may eventually add to the overall side effect burden.

Having taken these considerations into account, a change in medication may be the best option, in which case it is usually best to follow a personal prescribing algorithm. We discuss this in Chapter 13. The point here is that changes need to be logical and rational rather than random and hopeful. This does not necessarily mean invariably following guidelines and published evidence, as these are not the only source of guidance to rational practice. Some years ago a colleague mentioned to us that he had an inpatient who was suffering from severe extrapyramidal side effects due to a depot neuroleptic. He had decided to change the medication to oral quetiapine, which has to be dose-titrated in order to avoid hypotension and sedation. As it was likely to take weeks for the depot medication to clear from the patient's system he was not expecting any improvement in the immediate future. He was surprised to find that the side effects disappeared within twenty-four hours of commencing a low starting dose of quetiapine. We have subsequently found that a small dose of quetiapine (25 mg bd) can be remarkably effective in suppressing extrapyramidal side effects of neuroleptics where antimuscarinics fail or are contraindicated. It does not always work; it is not a licensed indication for quetiapine and it is not the strategy of choice. It does have the advantage of being safe and is a useful option in dealing with a troublesome side effect. Unconventional approaches to side effects can be productive, but have to be followed with caution, which means making the status of the treatment clear to the patient.

Depot antipsychotics

Psychiatrists in the UK were heavy prescribers of depot medication from the time that they became available, but depot injections were never as prominent in psychiatric practice in the USA. In recent years, things have changed. There is a body of opinion in the USA that is enthusiastic about the advantages of depot risperidone (Kane *et al.*, 2003), whilst UK practice has shifted away from the blanket use of depot medication to treat schizophrenia. Older mental health professionals and patients have bad memories of large depot clinics, attended by an over-medicated and neglected clientele. The advent of atypical antipsychotics, with claims of better tolerability and therefore better treatment adherence, certainly had an impact in reducing the use of the old depot drugs, which were potent dopamine blockers with an attendant high rate of movement side effects. However, it is likely that changes in attitudes about the relationship between services and patients had an equal effect in reducing the popularity of depot treatments.

There is no doubt that depot medications can be used coercively. The unwilling patient is started on a depot during a hospital admission. On discharge, the CMHT knows as soon as the patient declines to take the medication. It cannot be concealed because the depot is administered by a nurse. This is a strategy for monitoring treatment adherence, but it is one that dictates continued conflict, with little opportunity to move the relationship towards something that could realistically be described as therapeutic. However, the use of depot medication is not necessarily coercive. Indeed, the evidence suggests that patients who take depot long term have a positive attitude to the treatment. This echoes the debates and evidence over depot hormone contraception, which was highly controversial when it was introduced.

Patients recognise that they can inadvertently stop medication, and choosing to take a depot is one way of avoiding this. People forget to take tablets. They forget to order them from the pharmacist when their supply runs out. People suffer from stomach upsets that can make it impossible to keep tablets down. People can realise that they have not packed their medicine when they arrive at a foreign holiday destination. Unfortunately, notwithstanding our earlier comments about intermittent dosage schedules, some people's illnesses start to relapse after just a few days without medication. Having started to become ill, they can lose the awareness that they need to resume treatment. Depot medication is a sensible choice for some people and a surprisingly large number choose it if it is offered. It is unfortunate that we tend to suggest depot infrequently these days. However, there are many other ways of avoiding inadvertent discontinuation, ranging from daily telephone prompting to Post-it notes on the bathroom mirror.

Self-management strategies

It has always been evident that patients who learn to manage their illnesses are more likely to truly recover than those who do not. The service user movement has led the way in organising courses for people to develop self-management skills. These courses are important, but self-management strategies have wider implications, which are most clearly seen in the example of bipolar affective disorder.

The manifestations of bipolar affective disorder are intrinsically intermittent, and the idea that one should only take medication when it is necessary is attractive. On top of this, psychotropic medication can have the unfortunate effect of making things worse rather than better. Abrupt cessation of lithium carbonate can provoke a manic relapse. Antidepressants can induce mania. Antipsychotics can induce a stable but depressed mood. Although prophylaxis works well for some people, mood stabilisers do not work for a proportion of patients.

The alternative is to help patients to recognise their personal relapse signature. For most people there are certain situations and stressors that are especially likely to make them unwell, and there are particular key early warning signs, such as sleeplessness, that reliably augur relapse. Recognising these factors allows the patient to take action to avoid potent stressors and to initiate treatment in order to avoid a relapse. There is a general, though not invariable, rule that depressive episodes in bipolar affective disorder immediately follow manic episodes. If mood upswings are prevented, downswings tend not to occur. A typical plan would involve the patient holding a supply of an antipsychotic drug. They can start the medication without reference to a doctor whenever early warning signs are present, or even just to cover stressful periods in their life. They are able to see their psychiatrist or a member of the CMHT on request. This can take some days to arrange, so it is important that they should not have to wait before initiating treatment.

Plans such as these can work very well, but there are some pitfalls. People who have only had one or two episodes can find it difficult to identify early warning signs. This can mean that, in the process of learning about their illness, they experience several potentially avoidable episodes before the strategy starts to work. Mania can have a very rapid onset in some people, and by the time early warning signs are apparent, it is too late to avoid a full-blown episode. The course of bipolar affective disorder is in any case hard to predict, and it is difficult to give newly diagnosed patients guidance as to the likely outcome if they follow this strategy. The risks associated with disinhibition can be particularly difficult to evaluate after just one manic episode, which can make it difficult for the newly diagnosed patient to weigh the advantages and disadvantages of taking a chance on relapse. However, there is every reason to give patients this option amongst the range of available strategies. We are increasingly impressed with how well the approach can work. It must also be acknowledged that there are some types of patient for whom it does not work well: those who enjoy being manic, those who have severely unstable illnesses and those whose insight is very poor in the sense they cannot accept that they have a mental illness.

Specific interventions to achieve adherence

Cognitive behaviour therapies (CBTs) have found an increasingly prominent role in the treatment of mental illness, and it is not surprising that specific adherence therapy has emerged. The main characteristics of one form of adherence therapy are set out in Box 12.1.

It is immediately apparent that these are the same as the principles for achieving a good therapeutic alliance and adherence to treatment plans in general. There are strengths and weaknesses in developing this kind of therapy. CBT's ability to systematise treatment and to focus on what works are its great strengths. The weakness, however, is that it creates the temptation to take problems with the therapeutic alliance out of the therapeutic relationship. Adherence therapy is a tool to strengthen the therapeutic alliance. It is not a cure-all or an isolated intervention to fix a problem in the patient. It can only ever be an adjunct to the main task of getting alongside the patient.

Box 12.1 Adherence therapy (Gray *et al.*, 2006)

- Aims to achieve agreement about medication between individual and therapist through a brief individual CBT approach.
- Key elements include assessment and understanding medication history, exploration of beliefs, concerns and ambivalence about medication, problem solving, planning future medication use.
- The therapist exchanges information, works on resistance to discussion about psychiatric medication and treatment in order to draw out discrepancies between the subject's thoughts and behaviours.
- Depends on collaboration, flexibility and transparency.
- Therapist takes an active therapeutic stance, emphasises personal choice and responsibility, supports self-efficacy and improvements in self-esteem.

Pharmacists can play an important role with a mental health team. This includes providing patients with accurate and objective information on drugs. However, in our experience, this only works well if the pharmacist is a mental health specialist who has sufficiently close contact with the other mental health professionals so as to be regarded as part of the team. Without this, the information the pharmacist provides becomes de-contextualised and difficult to integrate with overall treatment plans. This is not to imply that psychiatrists need to control pharmacists in case they somehow become subversive. Just like adherence therapy, pharmacists' interventions have to be integrated into overall strategies in order to work.

Patients who do not take their medication are often referred to assertive outreach teams (AOTs). Assertiveness is a clinical stance aimed at overcoming problems with engagement. It is based on firm persistence and straight talking. It requires clinicians to maintain warmth and to continue with efforts to help patients through periods when they are resistant to some aspects of treatment. Assertiveness is not the same as duress, and it is not a tool to induce compliance. If the patient refuses medication because of non-engagement, then referral to an AOT can make a real difference. If the patient just does not agree with the treatment plan, then such a referral can make things worse, because it is immediately obvious that the AOT is being used as a 'heavy squad'. This is bound to make the patient suspicious of the AOT. It is far better, under these circumstances, that the current clinicians try to find a way through to agreement.

The bottom line

Much of this chapter has concerned people suffering from psychosis rather than non-psychotic illnesses such as depression, despite the fact that their rate of adherence to treatment is similar. The literature on concordance/compliance has the same skew. It seems to us that this is due to a crucial difference in our attitude towards people with these diagnoses. For whatever reason, we seem to be able to accept that people suffering from depression retain the right to make their own decisions (including the right to make mistakes). It is apparently harder for us to accept this when people are suffering from psychosis. When people lose the right to make bad decisions then they lose the right to make any decisions at all. For professionals to accept patients' autonomy and to work with their decisions is the difference between aiming at concordance and compliance. A willingness to continue to work with people who reject some part of your advice makes the difference between an impasse and a process of patient and clinician gradually coming together.

Finally, Professor Stefan Priebe and colleagues (2005), in a paper examining the reasons for disengagement from assertive outreach, point out that complaints about the effects of medication and loss of autonomy often turn on a single and negotiable issue. If such issues are addressed, it can be possible to develop a co-operative relationship, though this has implications for the quality of therapeutic relationships, including respect for people's need for independence.

Main points in this chapter

1. Treatment plans are adhered to better through agreement rather than through submission.
2. The illness belongs to the patient and it is his problem, not the doctor's.
3. Patients resist treatment for salient and understandable reasons.
4. Non-compliance is always an option, but mostly people want to be well.
5. Side effects can be managed without repeated changes of drug.
6. There is a range of strategies available to avoid relapse, from depot injections to intermittent medication, but the choice is the patient's.
7. Specific interventions to improve adherence have a role, but they are essentially adjunctive.

13 Treatment resistance

Much of the work of psychiatrists involves trying to help people suffering from illnesses that prove to be resistant to ordinary treatment. When patients get better quickly and easily, they do not spend much time with clinicians, so dealing with the problems associated with treatment resistance is a major part of the work of mental health services.

These days there are evidence-based guidelines that set out rational paths of treatment progression in resistant (or refractory) disorders. They are helpful, particularly as it has become increasingly difficult for jobbing clinicians to keep abreast of a rapidly expanding evidence base. However, guidelines have limited application, because they can only ever take into account one of the three arms of the 'triangle of forces', namely the technical. They are based on research that, in order to be scientifically valid, excludes many of the complicating problems that are common in daily clinical practice. Applying research findings is often difficult because the constraints of research create gaps and differences with clinical practice. Consequently, the preparation of guidelines involves the use of expert opinion and a degree of interpretation in moving from evidence to guidance. Guidelines are helpful, but they cannot be relied upon to provide all the answers.

There is a significant difference between the clinical problem of treatment resistance and the research concept of treatment refractory or resistant disorders. In research, it is important to have tight definitions and homogenous groups of subjects. Research criteria attempt to ensure that, in order to qualify as 'treatment resistant', the patient must have been exposed to a specified number of standard treatments pursued with sufficient vigour for an adequate time. In clinical practice, treatment resistance means the situation where the patient has received treatment but does not get better, and the clinician has to start to think about alternatives; it is also known as *getting stuck*. Treatment resistance, so defined, is a perception belonging to the clinician that can arise in a range of different situations. Managing treatment resistance often takes clinicians beyond the licensed indications for drugs, and into territory where there is no clear evidence to fall back on, which means that they need to avoid the pitfalls of irrational and chaotic treatment.

Factors associated with treatment resistance

Clinical treatment resistance is heterogeneous and, for the most part, partial. One does come across situations where a patient seems to be suffering from a condition that is truly refractory to treatment, but in our experience these situations are uncommon. When a patient is not improving and you feel stuck, it is important to try to exclude the common reasons that account for this. The main factors are:

- *Failure to obtain a full history.* We are veterans of countless case conferences, which frequently focus on a failure to get better. In a high proportion of such presentations it becomes apparent that there are significant gaps in the available history. This rarely seems to have arisen through carelessness. Often the patient has had their first contact with mental health services in a crisis, whereby they are severely unwell and are admitted to hospital. They are unable to give a full history at this stage, and the task then gets lost against the more pressing demands of dealing with the immediate situation and the vagaries of events. Sometimes close examination of a competent history reveals gaps where important information has been withheld, often flagged by a gap in the chronology. Sometimes important aspects of a 'well-known' patient's history have been forgotten, buried in the case notes and outside of the awareness of professionals who have been working with them for years. The starting point in all cases of treatment resistance has to be 'Have we got a comprehensive and accurate history?'

- *Wrong diagnosis/formulation.* All clinicians from time to time arrive at an erroneous or incomplete understanding of a patient's problems despite comprehensive assessment. Missing an underlying organic disorder is an example. Misinterpreting clinical features is another. Agitated depression is easily mistaken for an anxiety state due to personality problems. The unstable mood of borderline personality disorder can easily be mistaken for bipolar affective disorder. Intellectual impairment can lead to a variety of unusual presentations of anxiety and depression, but can go undetected if the person has good verbal skills. If treatment is not working, is it because it is the wrong type of treatment? We have pointed out elsewhere that diagnosis and formulation are always hypotheses, and one needs to review the strength of the evidence for and against them from time to time. This allows the psychiatrist to be careful and self-critical without sliding into indecisiveness and diagnostic instability.

- *Lack of clear or appropriate treatment objectives.* Sometimes failure to share treatment objectives means that symptomatic improvement does not bring about the change that is important to the patient. This can be due to contextual problems or complicating factors that frustrate progress. For example, a middle-aged woman presents with moderately severe depression against the background of alcohol misuse. With some help she stops drinking, but she substitutes cannabis for alcohol. She takes antidepressant medication and at interview her mood appears to have improved. However, she complains that she feels no better. She has been irritable from the outset and it emerges that she still is. This is causing major problems in her marriage. Coping with her irritability has always been a high priority for her. The psychiatrist had expected her irritability to resolve as her depression improved, but in fact cannabis has sustained it. For the psychiatrist, she has improved. For the patient she has not, because her most pressing problem has not resolved, and she does not recognise that, although cannabis has facilitated her abstinence from alcohol, it has worsened her irritability.

- *Inadequate treatment.* Psychiatrists have a low threshold of suspicion that the patient is covertly avoiding treatment. This is indeed a significant reason for failure to improve, and the range of techniques that people devise to avoid treatment is truly a testament to human ingenuity. However, it is by no means the only reason for inadequate treatment. There are real pressures on clinicians to get people better quickly, especially during inpatient admissions, and this can lead to the abandonment of treatments before they have had a chance to work. The entirely appropriate attention paid to patient choice can drive repeated changes of medication with similar results (in which case a part of helping the patient to make choices is making sure they understand that duration of treatment is a critical factor). A significant part of the work of tertiary referral centres involves making sure that standard treatments have been used adequately. In many cases clinicians think that they have pursued such strategies to the point that they have failed, but on careful examination of the records it turns out that they have not. If medication has not worked, you need to check the actual records (whether GP prescription records or inpatient drug charts) to see what has actually been prescribed.
- *Anti-therapeutic factors.* All mental health professionals are aware that substance misuse can impede improvement. For example, significant alcohol intake can nullify the effects of antidepressant medication, and it can exacerbate psychotic symptoms. More subtle anti-therapeutic factors can have an equally powerful effect. For example, when people are recovering from mania, quite ordinary amounts of stimulation can prevent the episode from resolving. Day leave from an inpatient unit or constant visits by friends can have this effect, which is problematic because it is entirely reasonable for the patient to want these things.
- *Treatment intolerance.* People vary enormously in the extent to which they suffer from side effects of medication, and in the degree to which they can tolerate them. A small but significant sub-group of people seem to get intolerable side effects from all medications, and although some of them are communicating their emotional resistance to taking medication, in many cases there does seem to be a real problem. Treatment intolerance frequently drives serial changes and treatment failure. The points in Chapter 12 regarding strategies to minimise side effects are relevant in avoiding this situation.
- *Disorders that exist outside of the standard nosology.* No matter how long you practise psychiatry, you continue to see people suffering from problems that you have never seen before and that do not conform to standard classification systems. These sometimes involve unusual combinations of symptoms, for example, distressing complex multimodality hallucinatory experiences associated with religious preoccupation in the absence of clear evidence of either schizophrenia or major affective disorder. Sometimes the clinical picture is dominated by psychopathology that does not correspond with any recognised phenomena, for example, transient episodes of severe, unfocussed anxiety with disinhibited, aggressive behaviour in the absence of convincing precipitants. Most clinicians tend to treat such conditions as if they were the disorder that the presentation most resembles. This can work, but sometimes it does

not, in which case a complete rethink may be more fruitful than a progression through a variety of treatments for the standard disorder.

- *Conditions that are intrinsically difficult to treat.* Some disorders simply do not respond well to any treatment. This is true of a proportion of cases of chronic and severe obsessive-compulsive disorder and of persistent delusional disorder (true paranoia). Poor prognosis disorders create a real dilemma with regard to the extent that one should accept that symptomatic change is unlikely. One is caught between the twin dangers of striving too hard to achieve the unachievable and neglecting the patient. The problem is that some patients do eventually improve, but other people do much better if one helps them to cope with symptoms rather than trying to eliminate them. Another group of people seem to do better without any intervention at all.

In what way is this disorder treatment resistant?

The next step that we have found helpful when we are feeling stuck is to think about the way in which the disorder is treatment resistant. In our experience very few people show no response to treatment. Even when you feel stuck, most patients have shown either a limited improvement or have got worse. We recognise six main types of treatment failure:

1. The patient improves, but not enough.
2. They improve, but recurrently rapidly relapse.
3. They move between different types of mental state abnormality.
4. Their mental state improves, but their behaviour does not.
5. Treatment appears to make them worse.
6. They truly show no response to treatment of any sort, and their condition is static.

Clearly each of these problems has a different type of solution and guidelines on managing treatment resistant disorders only deal with some of them. It is important to recognise which type of treatment failure you are dealing with. For example, rapid cycling bipolar affective disorder falls into type 3, but it is a term that is sometimes applied to patients with problems that fall into type 2. These problems have different origins, and it is fruitless to search, for example, for a more effective mood stabilising strategy, if some other difficulty, such as not taking medication or drinking heavily, is actually negating an effective treatment. In clinical practice, overcoming these problems requires analytical thinking, planning, a good understanding of the science and a degree of creativity.

Two clinical problems and their resolution

It is apparent from the above that, in our opinion, the key to managing situations that are stuck lies in the way you think about them. It is perhaps useful to give this some flesh through two somewhat different clinical vignettes. We do not recommend these as examples of ideal management, and we certainly do not offer the treatment plans as

---

Box 13.1 Treatment-resistant schizophrenia

Joseph was a forty-year-old single man who lived alone in a small housing association flat. He had first been admitted to hospital twenty years earlier, suffering from a schizophrenic illness. For many years he lived with his parents, until they became frail. He had recently moved into sheltered housing.

Following his first episode of illness, Joseph had never been free of psychotic symptoms. He believed that a man who had bullied him at school was organising a gang to kill him. If he avoided going out his symptoms were tolerable, a low muttering of auditory hallucinations. However, even trips to the corner shop made him anxious, and then the voices became loud, distracting and threatening. When he lived with his parents he rarely went out. Now that he was living alone he could not avoid regular visits to the town centre, and he coped by drinking. This calmed his nerves but it also caused an escalation of symptoms. He had been taking a depot antipsychotic for many years, which he felt was helpful to him. However, when his symptoms were severe, he was too fearful to answer the door, and his community mental health nurse was unable to give him his injection. The combination of unresolved symptoms, fearfulness, drinking and reclusiveness drove a cycle of relapse and hospitalisation.

From the point of view of the CMHT, Joseph's illness seemed to have seriously destabilised since he had been living alone. Initially the CMHT attributed this to the development of an alcohol problem, and its efforts were focussed on helping him to stay sober. He did sometimes become abstinent for a few weeks, but eventually his will would break, because he had no alternative strategy to cope with his anxiety. The net effect on the pattern of admissions was zero.

On re-evaluating the situation, the CMHT realised that although the pattern of recurrent admissions was new, Joseph's symptoms had never shown a good response to treatment. They had been a constant over two decades. The CMHT thought it might be possible to improve his well being if the symptoms could be reduced, and decided to try two interventions, namely CBT and a change to an oral atypical antipsychotic. Joseph would not engage in CBT, because he feared that he might give something away that his persecutor would use against him. He was forgetful with regard to his tablets. His symptoms worsened rather than improved.

At this stage there seemed to be little option but to admit him to hospital to ensure a proper trial of an atypical antipsychotic and, if this failed, to start him on clozapine. In truth, the psychiatrist and the community mental health nurse were certain that clozapine was the only thing that would make a difference. In their experience, clozapine was most often useful where there were active symptoms of psychosis. In other situations, for example prominent 'negative symptoms' or recurrent relapse, its effects were more disappointing. Sure enough, after four weeks on a standard dose of the new antipsychotic, Joseph was no better, and he was keen to try clozapine.

The effects of the clozapine were striking. After three weeks Joseph reported that the voices had stopped, and although he was still frightened of his persecutor, it was easier to put this out of his mind. He went home amid the high expectation of a better future. Everyone commented on how much better Joseph seemed. There were no further admissions. He remembered to take his tablets. He did complain that, although the background mumbling had stopped, he still heard frightening voices when he went out. He started to drink again to cope with this. He complained bitterly about weight gain. He could not be persuaded that this might be due to beer rather than medication because, as he pointed out, he had often drunk heavily in the past and he had never got fat before.

Eventually, he surprised the psychiatrist and the community mental health nurse by asking if he could go back on to the depot. It emerged that he had been thinking about this for sometime. He felt that, whilst the voices had improved, what with the side effects and everything else, overall he felt worse. The professionals were forced to recognise that the improvement in symptoms had failed to improve Joseph's sense of well being. At this point, the community mental health nurse made a radical suggestion. It appeared that anxiety was the main factor that drove Joseph's symptoms and his drinking. As psychological intervention had failed, why not go back to the depot as he requested and add a small regular dose of lorazepam?

There were many problems with this idea. Lorazepam is addictive, prone to misuse and has a potentially lethal interaction with alcohol. All guidance recommends that the drug should only be used short term, and this was a long-term strategy. Lorazepam is not a recognised treatment for schizophrenia (Volz *et al.*, 2007). It might be hard to get Joseph to understand the risks in order to give informed consent. It took several weeks to work through these issues with Joseph and to put plans in place in case things went wrong, particularly with regard to his drinking. In the end, however, the plan worked. Lorazepam did contain his anxiety, and his drinking remained under control. The voices finally disappeared. He became involved in a work scheme. Notwithstanding the unconventional nature of the treatment, Joseph was pleased with the improvement in his life.

models for others to follow. We do believe that they illuminate the process of finding a way through difficult clinical problems.

The main points that the story in Box 13.1 illustrates are:

- People who experience a poor outcome from treatment can easily go unnoticed when their behaviour causes little concern.
- Not only was the patient struggling with treatment-resistant symptoms, but there were also situational factors that contributed to the problem.
- The mental health team resisted the temptation of repetitively pursuing a strategy that had failed, i.e. trying to directly intervene with regard to Joseph's drinking.
- The team followed a conventional strategy, in keeping with national guidelines (National Institute for Clinical Excellence, 2002) until this proved unsuccessful. When the team followed an unconventional strategy it did so with a proper awareness of the pitfalls.

Box 13.2 Treatment-resistant depression

Derek was a sixty-three-year-old retired businessman who had suffered several episodes of depression since his mid-thirties. In the past he had been successfully treated by an office-based psychiatrist who had prescribed a tricyclic antidepressant. He had stayed on this drug for some years. He took retirement at the age of sixty. He and his wife intended to travel, but their plans were thwarted when he had a minor cerebrovascular accident. He made a full recovery but his confidence was permanently undermined by a new sense of physical vulnerability. His antidepressant was stopped with no ill effect whilst he was in hospital after the stroke.

Derek was admitted to his local psychiatric unit in a severely agitated state one Saturday afternoon. His wife had noticed that he was subdued for about three weeks, but she had been alarmed on the day of admission when he had become distraught. He sobbed as he confessed to her that he thought that he had given her a venereal disease as a result of a sexual indiscretion in his teens. All efforts to calm him failed, and a visit by the on-call GP led to referral to hospital.

On assessment, Derek was found to be suffering from a severe agitated depression. His guilty preoccupation over venereal disease appeared delusional. He was commenced on a standard dose of an SSRI, fluoxetine. His agitation worsened, and he constantly paced. After a few days, a modest dose of an atypical antipsychotic, quetiapine, was added in the hope that this might reduce his agitation and the intensity of his guilty preoccupations.

When the psychiatrist reviewed him he raised the possibility that Derek might be right and that his depression and his stroke might be due to untreated syphilis. Full physical investigations were arranged to exclude this and other organic factors. It was recognised that the clinical presentation had some features that would suggest a good response to ECT. The idea was held in reserve in case there was a poor response to other treatments.

During the first three weeks of inpatient treatment Derek's condition deteriorated. The dose of fluoxetine was increased, but his agitation worsened. Although it was, strictly speaking, too soon to say that fluoxetine had failed, the deterioration in his condition seemed ominous. The team planned a strategy in the expectation that Derek's condition was likely to prove difficult to treat.

Although management rested primarily on biological treatments, the team decided that a community mental health nurse should work with Derek's wife. It was likely that the situation was going to have a serious impact on her. The team needed a rational pathway that they could follow in the event that successive treatments failed. They decided to change fluoxetine to a tricyclic. They chose amitriptyline because, although it is an old drug, there is some evidence that it may be more effective than newer tricyclics. If this failed they planned to add lithium carbonate. Lithium augmentation enhances the effect of tricyclics and SSRIs. The team was anxious about giving two potentially toxic drugs, but this seemed reasonably safe in the hospital setting. If this failed, they would recommend a course of ECT.

The team intended to manage Derek's agitation with quetiapine, and expected his guilty worries to resolve as his mood improved. The team explained the plan in detail to Derek and his wife, and gave them some reading material about ECT.

The team's apprehensions proved well founded. They proceeded as planned, but Derek showed little sign of improvement. The admission dragged on, and by the time a course of ECT was started, Derek had been in hospital for ten weeks. He and his wife were anxious about the treatment, but they were prepared to go ahead. After four treatments, Derek was definitely less depressed, but progress stalled. After eight treatments he was much the same. After twelve treatments, everyone agreed that ECT should stop.

Derek had now sufficiently improved to be treated at home, but he was still far from well. He was gloomy and anxious, and he had no self-confidence. He could not drive his car, and he was reluctant to go out alone. He still had guilty worries, though they no longer had a delusional quality. He was taking amitryptiline, lithium and quetiapine.

The psychiatrist told Derek and his wife that he was reluctant to make further changes to Derek's medication. Whilst he could not exclude the possibility that another regime might work better, it seemed to him that biological treatment had achieved all that it could, and now they should try a different tack. He suggested CBT combined with a graded schedule of activity. Over the following year Derek slowly recovered. CBT helped him with his agitation and his guilty worries, and the graded activity, organised by a support worker, rebuilt some of his damaged self-confidence.

Eighteen months after he had been admitted, Derek had not returned to his former self. The ordeal of a protracted episode of mental illness exacerbated his sense of vulnerability following the stroke, and he was altogether a more anxious person than he had been. However, he functioned quite well day by day. He started driving his car again. Eventually the couple had their foreign holiday.

- A better outcome was achieved because the team accepted that the patient is the final arbiter of success or failure.
  The main points that the story in Box 13.2 illustrates are:
- Rather than exhausting all possible treatments, the team set out a strategy for managing treatment resistance at an early stage.
- This was shared with the patient and his wife, which helped to avoid despair as the admission dragged on.
- By setting realistic limitations to the likely effects of biological treatments, it was possible to continue to make progress, rather than getting locked in a continued search for a better response to drugs.
- Nothing in this case worked very well, but by adopting a rehabilitation approach, the patient did experience a type of recovery.
- CBT played a part. There is a tendency to look to CBT when all else has failed, and it is not surprising to find that it tends to disappoint under these circumstances. In our

experience, CBT works best in the treatment of serious mental illness when it is an integrated component of a wider plan.

Developing a personal prescribing algorithm

A theme of this book is the use of scientific evidence and clinical experience together to create strategies that are rational, safe and effective. As far as prescribing is concerned, this requires a type of internalised algorithm that creates a habitual pathway to follow when successive medications prove ineffective or hard to tolerate. Sometimes this algorithm is identical to a published guideline, such as can found in *The Maudsley Prescribing Guidelines* (Taylor *et al.*, 2007), but often experience leads you to make modifications. The task of establishing and maintaining such algorithms is an active and continuous one, and it requires a degree of self-discipline and organisation. If you change some part of the algorithm, you need to know why you are doing so. The only way that clinical experience can constructively guide the process is by making changes systematically. One can make some judgements about a new drug if you use it under similar circumstances with twenty patients. You can make no reliable judgements from experience with one patient.

Maintaining a personal algorithm involves a degree of skepticism over new treatments, but it also demands that existing practices should be examined with a critical eye. Thirty years ago, UK psychiatrists routinely used extremely high doses of antipsychotic medication in the treatment of both schizophrenia and mania. A starting dose of chlorpromazine 200 mg four times a day was regarded as entirely satisfactory, and many patients were given 500 mg four times a day. It is sobering to remember that we personally presided over such regimes, as did everybody else at the time. The change to lower and safer prescribing schedules came about as a consequence of clinicians becoming uneasy about serious side effects and through noticing that low doses worked as well as high ones.

By critically examining one's own experience and applying strategies in a systematic way, you can arrive at an algorithm that is robust under most, but not all, circumstances. Each of us has a different algorithm for the routine treatment of severe depression. One of these was followed in the case in Box 13.2. Here it is, with its rationale:

1. The first line antidepressant is fluoxetine 20 mg/day. It has a long half-life, which tends to minimise withdrawal effects, but otherwise it is no better or worse than other SSRIs. However, it is a very familiar drug, and in the absence of a more effective medication, there is no reason to stop using it.
2. If the pattern of symptoms (mainly sleeplessness and agitation) or previous response suggest that a tricyclic might be more appropriate, use amitryptiline 150 mg/day instead. The choice of amitryptiline is influenced both by familiarity and by evidence suggesting that it may be somewhat more effective than other antidepressants.
3. Mirtazepine 30 mg/day can be used if a sedative effect at night seems desirable and there is a good reason not to use amitryptiline.
4. If there is no response or a partial response to an antidepressant, the dose can be adjusted once, to a maximum of fluoxetine 40 mg/day or amitryptiline 200 mg/day.

5. If this fails, reduce to standard dose and add lithium carbonate. Aim for a blood level at the low end of the therapeutic range, because this minimises side effects and does not seem to compromise effectiveness. This augmentation strategy is well tolerated and has a high rate of success.
6. If lithium augmentation fails, consider ECT.

Naturally, there are a number of circumstances that can make it necessary to use other drugs, but such algorithms can be adhered to most of the time. This algorithm positively excludes some potential strategies:

- Combinations of antidepressants from different classes, because any supposed advantage in effectiveness seems to be outweighed by the burden of combined side effects.
- High dose antidepressants. At one time venlafaxine had a place in the algorithm, including higher doses (200 mg/day plus), but it was dropped because of the high rate of side effects. Lithium augmentation seems to be both more effective than this and carries a lower side effect burden.
- Non-antidepressant drug strategies such as thyroxin and anticonvulsant mood stabilisers, owing to a lack of evidence that they reliably work.

No doubt many experienced psychiatrists would disagree with this algorithm and would be able to make cogent criticisms of it which we would not deny. We do not believe that it is desirable to include every respectable treatment that is available. The point of the exercise is not the detail. The point is to have a schema that works most of the time without undue side effects and that allows a timely movement through treatments, of increasing potency. This brings coherence and structure to treatment and avoids the situation where you find yourself flicking through the British National Formulary, wondering what to do next.

The use of combinations of drugs is a particularly difficult issue. There is a general consensus that polypharmacy is a bad thing, to be avoided wherever possible, though there is a small body of opinion within psychopharmacology that suggests it might be possible to make fine adjustments of neurotransmitter function by judicious use of combinations. We strongly favour the avoidance of drug combinations, but the one thing that is obvious about polypharmacy is that nearly all prescribers do it, including us. This being the case, is it really such a bad thing?

The evidence with regard to combinations of drugs is very limited compared with the much more extensive literature concerning the effects of individual drugs. It is self-evident that, generally speaking, the use of more than one drug in order to treat the same problem is bound to increase side effects, and we have never been impressed by the effectiveness of combinations of antipsychotics or of antidepressants. However, there are some exceptions to the rule that polypharmacy is rarely better than monotherapy. For example, the combination of lithium with an anticonvulsant mood stabiliser often achieves effective prophylaxis in bipolar affective disorder where each fails on its own. There is a further good reason to avoid being excessively dogmatic about completely avoiding drug combinations. Psychotropic drugs treat symptoms, not diseases. Some patients have combinations of symptoms that are best controlled by drugs from different classes.

The role of the magical and dramatic in managing treatment resistance

Many years ago, long before clozapine became available, one of us had a patient with a severe schizophrenic illness that showed no response whatever to standard treatments. The severity of psychotic symptoms was such that conversation was near impossible. Hallucinatory voices were so intrusive that discussion constantly seemed three-way. After a year in hospital and the failure of a range of treatments, therapeutic hopelessness had set in and he was awaiting transfer to a long-stay rehabilitation ward. At this point, on the suggestion of a trainee, the consultant added carbamazepine. Within ten days the psychotic symptoms completely resolved. Over a long period of follow-up his illness appeared to respond completely to the combination of carbamazepine and an antipsychotic, but only to this combination.

Such a dramatic response is bound to have a big impact on the clinician, and it did. At one time or another carbamazepine has been recommended for the treatment of epilepsy, treatment-resistant schizophrenia, rapid cycling bipolar affective disorder, episodic dyscontrol syndrome and irritability related to brain injury. The psychiatrist in this case was aware of being drawn to a seductive thought: Why not try adding carbamazepine whenever treatment gets stuck, irrespective of diagnosis?

Gambling is sustained by intermittent reinforcement. The excitement of winning blinds the gambler to the fact that he is much more frequently losing. Exactly the same process can persuade a psychiatrist of the magical potency of a drug like carbamazepine. It does work in treatment-resistant psychosis, but only sometimes. It may have a role (we sometimes use it for prophylaxis in bipolar affective disorder, despite the current ascendancy of semisodium valproate), but like all one-size-fits-all solutions it fails more frequently. In our opinion, exactly the same is true of certain magical cocktails, for example clozapine plus one or another atypical, that some people strongly advocate in treating patients with clozapine-resistant schizophrenia. Taken overall, the blanket use of magical strategies is more of a hindrance than a help in managing treatment-resistant disorders.

It is nearly always true that treatments that take on a destructively magical quality do have some value, and sometimes perfectly respectable treatments can be unwittingly misused in this way. Transcranial magnetic stimulation (TMS) has generated interest for some years now, and it is sometimes construed as a benign alternative to ECT in depression. This means that it is tempting to refer patients for TMS when antidepressant drugs have failed, because ECT is usually the next step and TMS seems less alarming. However, whilst there is evidence that TMS may have a limited role in treating depression, it is entirely dissimilar to ECT. ECT is the single, most effective treatment for severe depression with biological features, especially where there are delusions. TMS, on the other hand, may be less effective than antidepressants, and there is little evidence regarding its role in treatment-resistant depression. TMS is something of a blind alley as a strategy to overcome treatment failure, but this is not to assert that it has no role at all. It is the magical quality that is unhelpful.

Similar processes can occur when referrals are made for psychological therapies because all other options have been exhausted. CBT, psychodynamic therapies, psychosocial interventions and so on all have a significant role to play, but they cannot work magically as a disconnected intervention of last resort. However, what can be helpful is a consultation with a professional outside of the team to help you to think differently about a problem. We expressed our misgivings about the usefulness of second opinions at the end of Chapter 5. We are not dismissive of the value of tertiary centres with special expertise, but do feel that they should be used sparingly and with a clear understanding of what it is they might be able to offer a particular patient. We are, on the other hand, firm believers in the importance of talking cases through properly, be it with colleagues or experts, in order to get a different perspective or, occasionally, to reassure yourself that you have done everything possible in the situation. Both consultations and second opinions tend to be most valuable where you are able to frame a clear question to be answered, not least because it helps you to get your own ideas in order.

Nasty and forbidden treatments

Some treatments have a bad reputation with the general public, with clinicians or with both. Treatments do not acquire such a reputation for no reason. ECT is a prime example. Most British psychiatrists regard ECT as safe and highly effective in the treatment of certain specific conditions, namely severe or psychotic depression, mania and catatonic states. It is used sparingly, but few general adult and old age psychiatrists in the UK avoid its use altogether. The weight of opinion in the USA is different, and the general public, by and large, abhor 'electric shock treatment'. It is sometimes said that ECT acquired its bad reputation because of the way it was depicted in the film *One Flew Over the Cuckoo's Nest*, but this is erroneous. The film reflected rather than led public opinion about the treatment.

In the 1950s and early 1960s ECT was used almost indiscriminately in UK mental hospitals. One of us had a relative who was given ECT for a schizophreniform episode in 1968, at which time it was already known that it was not effective in this condition. In the earlier part of this period it was given without muscle relaxant or anaesthetic (when the Royal College of Psychiatrists surveyed facilities in 1980, they found that unmodified ECT was still being used at a number of locations). Amongst the thousands of people who were given the treatment in the early days, there were undoubtedly some who benefited very considerably. It was probably life saving in cases of stuporose depression prior to the development of alternative treatments. However, because it was given indiscriminately and unmodified, for most people the treatment was dangerous, very unpleasant and largely ineffective. Unmodified ECT has an obvious resonance with the methods used by torturers. The view of the general public has its basis in reality, and it is hardly surprising to find that there is some skepticism that things have changed.

There is a dilemma here. ECT's reputation makes it inappropriate as a first-line treatment, because there are effective alternatives. The patient's realisation that you might contemplate using it can have an adverse effect on the therapeutic relationship. You have to respect this reputation because it affects the treatment's usefulness. Set against this is its unassailable effectiveness in depressions that are otherwise treatment resistant. When ECT seems necessary, you have to work with the perception that it is nasty, which takes time. Bland reassurances and pressure to accept the treatment are counter-productive. Most of all, we believe that the use of ECT under legal compulsion should be avoided under all but the most extreme circumstances.

The other really 'nasty' psychiatric treatment is psychosurgery. There has been a small resurgence of interest in its use in recent years. Where the evidence for the effectiveness of ECT is compelling, the evidence for psychosurgery is not. Neither of us has ever referred a patient for psychosurgery. Twenty-five years ago we treated many patients who had been given psychosurgery in the years following the Second World War. Few seemed to have benefited much, but they did not conform to the stereotype of the shuffling lobotomised zombie either. We are aware that modern techniques are safe, and that there are claims of excellent results for some conditions. In refusing to contemplate psychosurgery for our patients, are we being sensibly skeptical or are we indulging our squeamishness to the detriment of tormented patients with intractable illnesses? Frankly, we have no answer to this question.

There is a similar problem over the use of drugs that have developed a bad reputation amongst prescribers and hence have become 'forbidden'. Sometimes this is appropriate enough. Monoamine oxidase inhibitors (MAOIs) were not very effective and they were prone to abuse (some of these drugs had a marked amphetamine-like effect). There were dangerous interactions with other drugs and some foodstuffs. The newer, less troublesome reversible inhibitor of monoamine oxidase, moclobamide, has never really caught on, which probably says something about the usefulness of the entire class of drug. Few have lamented the disappearance of MAOIs from clinical practice.

The use of benzodiazepines tends to cause psychiatrists discomfort. Few doubt their importance in the management of acute disturbance in the inpatient setting, and they have a respectable role in the treatment of catatonic states, where antipsychotics are often ineffective or may even make the patient worse (Hawkins *et al.*, 1995). Prescribing them for outpatients, however, is quite another thing. These drugs are awesomely addictive, and well-meaning efforts to use them to ease the pains of everyday life could arguably be said to have sedated a generation of women. However, this does not mean they have no role in the management of anxiety, as was set out in Box 13.1. There is perhaps an inconsistency here with our attitude to psychosurgery, but nonetheless we believe that it is self-indulgent for clinicians to completely reject the use of benzodiazepines in the management of intractable anxiety because, provided you are attentive to the dangers, they can give some patients a peace of mind that cannot be achieved in any other way.

Intractably stuck

No matter what you do, sometimes treatment becomes intractably stuck. When the problem concerns the treatment of psychosis or severe depression during an inpatient admission, you have to recognise when you have failed. This often means that the patient has to be referred to a different team or to a different hospital. In our opinion, it is important from the outset of such a referral to think about how it fits into a longer term plan of treatment. Under most circumstances, it is most appropriate that the patient should be able to come back to your team when the other team has completed its work. A no-return referral away can make the patient feel that they have been spat out and written off. People who have been so unwell that a referral away has been necessary are likely to need long-term follow-up. In order to maintain a continuity and coherence in treatment, it is good practice for the team to retain some involvement in care planning for patients referred away, because this makes the return journey much easier.

There is an important alternative strategy that can be useful for patients in the community suffering from intractable symptoms. It sometimes becomes apparent that there is no realistic possibility that symptoms are going to abate, because they have been present to a greater or lesser extent for decades or since childhood, and there is no evidence that a range of treatments has made any difference. Many such patients suffer from chronic anxiety and depression, or obsessional symptoms, and are seen by a succession of mental health professionals for many years, taking medication regimes that tend to be complex. Most of these patients know perfectly well that their symptoms are not going to go away. The professional also knows this, but is reluctant to say so, for fear of plunging patients into hopelessness. Patients take their leads from the professional in continuing to pursue strategies that differ only slightly from those that have already failed. They usually feel that they have little control over their lives, because they are hemmed in by symptoms and the methods they use to cope with them, by medication and by the unending need to see mental health professionals.

These stuck situations can sometimes be unstuck by acknowledging that the symptoms are unlikely to go away, and by changing the focus to helping patients to regain control of their lives. This means gradually withdrawing medications to see if they are necessary (sometimes they are, often they are not). Many patients feel much better about themselves if they can stop medication, even when symptoms persist. Treatment becomes a process of looking at what people can do despite symptoms, and of helping them to develop coping strategies to increase the range of things they can do.

This takes time and effort, and is usually only possible when a new professional becomes involved. However, it can work very well provided you do not mislead yourself or patients that it is possible that it will result in symptoms abating. It rarely does. However, patients can get better lives, and this is a type of recovery.

Conclusion

At this stage, some readers will be feeling cheated, because we have not set out any specific strategies for treatment-resistant disorders. The evidence with regard to the optimal management of treatment-resistant disorders changes all the time, and it is easy enough to access. However, we have found that the ability to think around problems of treatment resistance is just as important as knowledge of specific treatments.

We have explored situations here that do not strictly qualify as treatment resistance. We strongly believe that there is a continuity between common problems of lack of response and the rarer difficulties associated with unremitting severe illness. We do not think that it is helpful to regard treatment-resistant disorders as a separate and different type of problem, because they are not. To regard them as such tends to lead to therapeutic despair and plans that focus exclusively on physical treatments.

Two points seem to us to be particularly important and worth reiterating. Firstly, when patients do not get better, it is rarely solely due to the nature of the illness itself. There are usually emotional, environmental or situational factors that are contributing to the situation. They deserve attention. Secondly, treatments take time to work. Therapeutic impatience can lead to unnecessarily high doses of medication. It can be a cause of treatment failure, because the clinician moves on to the next treatment before the current one has had time to work.

Main points in this chapter

1. There are a number of different types of treatment failure, each of which has a different type of solution.
2. Treatment failure is rarely due solely to the intrinsic nature of the illness.
3. Having a personal prescribing algorithm helps to keep changes in treatment structured and coherent when the patient does not respond well.
4. It is difficult to avoid polypharmacy altogether, but the routine use of multiple drugs for the same indication is a bad habit.
5. Magic treatments and magical cocktails may appear to consistently work, but they do not. What makes things complicated is that they do work sometimes.
6. Some treatments are regarded as either seriously nasty or as forbidden. You may still need to use them, but you have to have respect for their nasty or forbidden status.
7. When the situation is intractably stuck, it is not very constructive to get rid of the patient by referral or to officiously strive to achieve the impossible. There are other alternatives.

14 Complicated problems

If a large part of a psychiatrist's work concerns treatment resistance, then much of the rest of it involves complicated problems. Sometimes you see a new patient and it becomes clear that he is suffering from a typical and common pattern of symptoms. This leads you to a diagnosis, which in turn determines a simple intervention. The patient adheres to a treatment plan, and recovers. This uncomplicated progression of assessment–diagnosis–treatment–recovery has not characterised very much of our work in the course of our professional lives, and we suspect this is true for most psychiatrists. Much more often there is a recognisable illness but there is also a variety of contextual problems and stresses, some of which have to be dealt with in order for the patient to get better, and some of which resolve as a result of successfully treating the illness. For the most part, these contextual difficulties are embedded in the overall situation. They are not separate from the illness; they are an intrinsic aspect of being mentally unwell for this particular person.

Some types of contextual difficulties have such a powerful effect in preventing improvement and recovery that they have to be regarded as major complicating factors, and they demand as much attention as the primary problem. The most prominent of these complications is substance misuse. The combination of psychosis and substance misuse has come to be known as 'dual diagnosis' and in many areas there are specialist dual diagnosis teams. We do not like the term very much. There are other dualities of diagnosis that are important in psychiatry, such as psychosis and learning disability. More importantly, it is far from clear that it is correct to regard substance misuse as a co-morbidity with psychosis. Most studies suggest that 25–50% of people suffering from bipolar disorder or schizophrenia have problems with substance misuse, which is considerably higher than the figure for the general population (e.g. McCreadie, 2002). It is probably more accurate to regard a vulnerability to substance misuse as part of the illness syndromes rather than as a separate problem.

Whether or not one regards major complicating factors as intrinsic to or distinct from the primary problem, they have to be dealt with, though it is the nature of things that this is rarely easy. The biggest pitfall lies in regarding patients with a complicating difficulty as somebody else's problem. One of the main reasons for the establishment of dual diagnosis teams has been the common pattern whereby nobody wants to treat such patients. Drug and alcohol teams complain that they are too mentally unwell for them, and CMHTs complain that their interventions cannot work whilst the patient is misusing substances. This is hard to defend. In our experience, the problems caused by substance misuse can usually be managed within an ordinary CMHT if it is willing to try to do so, and this is equally true of most other major complicating factors (Mental Health Policy Implementation Guide, 2002).

Substance misuse and psychosis

At present there is considerable excitement over the suggestion that heavy cannabis use in the early teenage years may combine with a genetic vulnerability to cause schizophrenia in some people. Opinions vary on the meaning of this work, but we are not going to explore it here, because it has no bearing on managing people with established psychosis. Suffice to say that the jury is still out on this matter.

All degrees of substance misuse can cause significant difficulties, from casual recreational use to committed addiction. The biggest problems arise when people adopt a lifestyle built around their habit. Committed substance misusers tend to hang about together, and they form small communities with a distinctive subculture. For example, there are knots of street drinkers huddled on benches in all city centres, and less visible networks of opiate and stimulant users who use run down flats to purchase and take drugs together. Although these subcultures are essentially deviant, they have major attractions for people who have become socially marginalised because of chronic psychotic illnesses. These communities are tolerant of socially inappropriate behaviour. They offer routines, companionship and a purpose. They can offer people with serious mental illness a sense of belonging and somewhere to be.

Set against this is the fact that, irrespective of the effects of drugs or alcohol per se, these lifestyles do not promote recovery from mental illness. They impede it. They put people outside of the law and in constant hostile contact with the authorities. They make it very difficult to secure adequate housing. These lifestyles cause physical ill health, poverty and a number of other serious problems that are inimicable to recovery from mental illness. Substance misusing subcultures are vortices, easy to get sucked into, but difficult to climb out of, even if you want to.

People with chronic psychosis living in these communities need help to develop a better life, because without this they cannot recover from their illness. Even if it is possible to simply secure them a nicer flat and a day centre to attend, it is futile, because nine times out of ten, the patients will soon drift back to their old lives. You have to understand the benefits to them of living this way, and try to find better ways of meeting the same needs. This invariably takes time.

Although committed substance misusers may have strong preferences with regard to drug of choice, and although drinkers and drug users are different to each other, most serious drug misuse involves poly-drug use. The standard international classification systems are unhelpful as they tend to classify psychological reactions substance by substance. On top of this, they assume that causality is easily determined, that is, that substances cause symptoms. A few years ago we attended a post-graduate psychiatric meeting where a case was being presented. There was a debate over whether the patient's psychotic symptoms were being caused by drug use or whether the patient was suffering from schizophrenia and the drug use was exacerbating this. One of our colleagues, an old age psychiatrist complained: 'I don't know why you general adult psychiatrists keep on presenting cases like this, because it always turns out that the patient has a mental illness and it never turns out that it's all down to the drugs.' We could only agree.

Despite attempts to eradicate the use of the term 'drug-induced psychosis' (i.e. a psychosis provoked by drugs that persists beyond intoxication) because there is little or no evidence that it exists, it will not die (Poole & Brabbins, 1996). There is continued confusion over the pharmacological impact of substance misuse on both the mentally well and the mentally ill. This has an adverse effect on patients, because there are often major delays in obtaining proper treatment because a drug problem complicating mental illness has been taken to be the sole cause of the patient's problems.

There is no point in pedantically listing the effects of individual substances, but we note that some drugs have little direct effect on symptoms of mental illness. Heroin misuse is a very bad thing, but it appears to be at worst neutral with respect to psychotic symptoms, and may even have a mildly antipsychotic effect. However, it is worthwhile reiterating the types of reactions that can occur, because they have some influence on the type of intervention that is appropriate:

- *Intoxication mimicking functional psychosis.* As is well known, high doses of amphetamine can cause schizophreniform symptoms that persist as long as the drug is in the body. This is what most people mean by 'drug-induced psychosis'. It also occurs with cocaine, but it is then short lived because cocaine has a very short half-life. What is confusing is that there appears to be a kindling effect. Having happened to you once, it tends to recur at progressively lower doses. When it occurs recurrently, it can be difficult to distinguish from schizophrenia complicated by drug use, but in fact the management is much the same in either case. Efforts to reduce or stop drug use are important, but antipsychotic medication will usually prevent these episodes, whether or not the person has an underlying mental illness.

- *Pathoplastic reactions.* Substance misuse can add to or shape symptoms of mental illness. Amongst the dose-dependent effects of cannabis on mentally well subjects are muddled thinking and paranoid anxiety. Consequently, when people who are hypomanic take cannabis, they can seem to be suffering from schizophrenia, because they appear disinhibited, thought disordered and paranoid. Similarly, it is not surprising that people suffering from acute schizophrenia deteriorate when the muddling, paranoid effects of cannabis are added to the effects of the illness. Most cannabis users say they take it because it makes them feel mellow and it helps them to chill out. However, the drug has an awesome ability to make people irritable. Cannabis has an extremely long half-life, and irritability tends to kick in as the relaxing effects wear off, an hour or two after consumption.

- *Chronic hallucinosis caused by substance misuse.* Hallucinogens, such as LSD and cannabis, can cause 'flashbacks' long after heavy use has stopped. Heavy alcohol use, sustained for years, routinely causes very unpleasant and vivid auditory hallucinations. The patient is aware that the hallucinations come from within himself, but often is unable resist shouting back at them. The hallucinations can also be visual. They start during intoxication and may persist through many months of abstinence before they finally fade. They recur very rapidly on re-exposure to alcohol, and may take just as long to fade again. They rarely respond at all to antipsychotic medication, which makes it very important to distinguish alcoholic hallucinosis from schizophrenia complicated by heavy drinking. In the latter, the patient's symptoms worsen and are more difficult to treat, but it is still worth prescribing antipsychotics, because people get worse still if you stop them. In alcoholic hallucinosis a trial of medication is worthwhile, but one usually stops it again, because it usually makes little difference.

- *Drug-induced relapse.* All psychiatrists recognise that cannabis misuse and heavy drinking commonly impede patients' recovery from all forms of mental illness. Some strongly believe that substance misuse can induce a relapse of mental illness despite continuing, and previously satisfactory, treatment. We once believed this, but we have come to doubt it. It appears to us that people often start drinking or misusing drugs when they are relapsing, and whilst this does not help matters, the substance misuse is more of a marker of relapse than a cause. One of the factors that has changed our mind is that we have found that it is more fruitful to treat the illness more vigorously than to concentrate too much on the substance misuse. It can be possible to avert the impending relapse in this way.

- *Withdrawal states.* Delirium tremens (DTs) is the severest of all withdrawal states, and whilst it is usually due to abrupt discontinuation of alcohol, it can also occur with other substances with anticonvulsant effects, such as benzodiazepines and barbiturates. It can occur unexpectedly when people are admitted to hospital, for example in people suffering from depression who have failed to disclose a heavy alcohol intake. One is sometimes called by inexperienced ward staff, who tell you 'He's gone psychotic!' DTs is a life-threatening medical emergency. Fortunately the condition looks very different to other psychiatric disorders, with severe restlessness, tremor, clouding of consciousness, fearfulness and a hallucinosis that causes an exaggerated behavioural response. The main point here is that one needs to maintain a high level of suspicion of DTs whenever a patient's mental state shows a dramatic, abrupt or unexpected shift towards 'psychosis' or confusion.

- *Intoxication leading to clouding of consciousness.* Another cause of a sudden unexpected deterioration in a patient's condition is a kind of delirium caused by drug use. This is rather uncommon with street drugs, and is more often associated with the use of large doses of prescription or over-the-counter medications. It is generally due to sedative effects and the most common example in our experience is the misuse of proprietary cough medicines, many of which have a hefty kick if taken in large quantities. The clue is the presence of a clouding of consciousness and other features of delirium. MDMA (ecstasy) is not sedative, but a handful of tablets taken in pursuit of friendship and fun can have the unwelcome effect of causing a delirious state with disorientation, impaired awareness of the environment, vivid visual and auditory hallucinations, and marked distress. Both people with mental illness and the more reckless kind of club attender can find themselves in hospital by this route. The condition tends to persist for several days, and although medication calms people down, it does not modify the course of the delirium.

- *Post-intoxication depression.* Stimulants cause a crash after the high, but the biggest problem is alcohol. It is a potent anxiolytic with an equally powerful capacity to cause post-intoxication depression. Consequently, all heavy drinkers are depressed to a greater or lesser extent. There is a marked impact on the mood of people with depressive illness. This occurs at quite modest doses, well within the range of 'normal social drinking'. Drinking is a common cause of depression in people with schizophrenia, and it is not surprising to find that heavy drinking destabilises bipolar affective disorder. In fact, taken over all, alcohol is by far the most troublesome substance of misuse that complicates the treatment of mental illness, both from the point of view of the range of its effects, and with regard to the proportion of people who take it (which in most patient populations is about double the number who misuse drugs). It is interesting to note that, whilst dual diagnosis has been the subject of many scientific publications in recent years, virtually nothing has been published about the interaction between alcohol and psychosis.

• *Panic due to intoxication.* People who dislike feeling out of control, which includes almost everyone with a significant degree of obsessionality in their personality, often suffer from panic attacks when they take hallucinogens such as LSD and cannabis. This does not merit much attention here, because by and large they only ever do it once.

Far too many patients misuse drugs and alcohol to make it practical to refer them all to specialist drug and alcohol services or dual diagnosis teams. In any case, even if it were possible, it would not be desirable. Specialist interventions for substance misuse depend on the motivation to stop. Many of our patients believe that their substance misuse is a part of the solution to their difficulties, and your job is to help them to see that it is a part of the problem. Once this is achieved, the task of overcoming substance misuse is easier. Some patients, such as the opiate addicted and the frankly alcoholic, do need help from specialist services as part of their treatment. These interventions usually work best through joint working, as opposed to serial intervention or parallel working. Both services need to be fully involved in treatment planning, and to have a close awareness of what the other is doing, in order to ensure that overall treatment is coherent. Ensuring that there are regular joint meetings involving the two teams and the patient is an important practical measure to achieve this.

Abstinence is invariably the ultimate objective when substance misuse complicates mental illness. This is not necessarily the case in the treatment of substance dependency. There is a good evidence for controlled drinking programmes, for example, but the effect of alcohol on mental illness is too pronounced to make it a sensible objective. However, abstinence is often a long time coming, and people need help with their mental illness in the meantime. Harm reduction can make a big difference, by changing the route by which drugs are taken or the quantities consumed or the choice of drugs. Harm reduction is about minimising the damage done rather than eliminating it.

To be effective you have to take a particular position over substance misuse. Patients have to feel that you understand drugs, alcohol, the subculture and the apparent benefits of their habits. This can only be achieved by talking with patients about their lifestyles in a non-judgemental way. Advice that substance misuse is having a bad effect is much easier to accept from someone who seems to understand and who is not critical when abstinence does not happen quickly. To do this it is not necessary to collude with continuing substance misuse. It is all about being clear and trying to work together to find a way forward. Anything that smacks of moralising is highly counter-productive.

The same principles are applicable to the management of all volitional behaviours that have an adverse effect on recovery from mental illness. We have dwelt on substance misuse at length because it is the most common of these problems.

Pregnancy and puerperium

Pregnancy and the perinatal period are an example of a complicating factor of a completely different type. What makes things difficult here, as in some other circumstances in clinical practice, is the involvement of two vulnerable people whose needs are different. On top of this, the involvement of a baby evokes an emotional reaction in the professionals that complicates everybody's thinking.

The most common scenario is where patients already under the care of the service either fall pregnant or are planning to get pregnant. If they suffer from a serious mental illness and medication is important to protect them from relapse, there is an immediate dilemma over the effect of the medication on a developing foetus. Following the thalidomide disaster, the universal and sound advice is to discontinue medications wherever possible, at least during the first trimester. The difficulty here is that the risks cannot be quantified and compared. Although some drugs are known to cause problems in foetuses, drugs are not tested on them, so the size of the risk is unclear. Thirty years ago it was said that lithium caused abnormalities in a high proportion of babies exposed to it in the first trimester. Whilst it is known that there is a problem with lithium, it is now believed that the proportion of affected babies is far lower, though it is difficult to derive a figure for risk that can easily be understood by the general public (Cohen *et al.*, 1994; Yonkers *et al.*, 2004). No one seems to know if blood level makes a difference. Furthermore, no one can say if other drugs are safer or not. Continuing medication may pose a teratogenic risk, but it may ensure that the mother remains well through pregnancy and the puerperium. Stopping medication may avoid exposure in the first trimester, but by provoking relapse may increase exposure to other drugs later in pregnancy, and may create the additional risk that the baby will be separated from the mother at birth in the event that she is ill at the time (Viguera *et al.*, 2000). Only God-like prescience could allow an accurate balancing of these risks, and yet the clinician has to find some way of weighing them with the patient and her family.

If, as is often the case, patients decide to continue with medication, they need to give some thought to the fact that there is always a risk that any child will be born with an abnormality (5% of all babies are born with some kind of problem). If an abnormality occurs, there is no way of knowing whether the drug caused the problem or not. This creates the potential for a lot of guilt, which may or may not be helped by forethought.

There is a range of medication strategies that can be deployed other than complete discontinuation, but they all have the disadvantage that they are based on common sense rather than clear evidence. They tend to be sub-optimal as far as avoiding relapse is concerned and it is hard to know to what extent they protect the baby. Discontinuation during the first trimester with resumption thereafter, changes from drugs that are known to cause problems to those where there is no data, dosage reductions and monotherapy in place of polypharmacy are examples of common sense but evidence-free strategies.

The bottom line is that these choices are for the mother to make, and one has to steer a path between the pitfalls of making the decision yourself (and trying to impose it) and completely befuddling the patient by presenting the information in a form that is confusing and overwhelming. This means you have take time, avoid pressing for a decision too fast and prevent yourself from conveying your anxieties over the ambiguities to the patient. Above all, you have to make the no-medication option a possibility, which means that the team may have to offer a greatly increased level of support during the pregnancy. This can be difficult when the patient adopts an unrealistically optimistic stance over either the risk of relapse without medication or the risk to the fœtus if it is continued. At the end of the day, these are stances that people have a right to take, and you have to help them deal with the consequences.

Anyone who has had personal experience of the process of giving birth and looking after a neonate knows that it is one of the most emotionally and physically stressful of human experiences. The fact that people like having babies does nothing to ameliorate this, because most people occasionally feel pretty negative towards their newborn baby and then feel guilty about it. Given the close relationship between stress and mental illness, it is no surprise that the puerperium is a time of high risk for relapse and for developing a mental illness de novo. Massive alterations in hormones may also play a role, but one suspects that it is a minor factor compared with everything else.

The last thing that either mother or child needs is for her to be mentally unwell after giving birth. Fortunately, one usually has plenty of time to plan to avoid a relapse. The issue of medication tends to loom large in psychiatrists' thinking, though it is not necessarily the most important or difficult issue. Of course, medication strategies do play a role. They involve close liaison with midwives to ensure, for example, discontinuation around the expected date of delivery (in order to avoid the baby having side effects after birth) and resumption in the immediate postnatal period. Medication during breastfeeding is less problematic than medication during pregnancy, because there are drugs that do not appear in breast milk. In any case, although bottle feeding is unfashionable and tiresome, it does not represent a major health risk to the baby.

There are other strategies that can protect mothers from postnatal relapse. Measures to ensure that the mother has adequate emotional and practical support are equally important as medication. Help to ensure that she gets rest and sleep, social contact, help to get the shopping in and so on can greatly reduce the degree to which the stress of the situation affects her mental health.

Psychiatrists are routinely summoned to pre-birth case conferences arranged by child protection agencies to decide whether the unborn child is at risk and if so, what should be done about it. In the section on liaising with external agencies in Chapter 6 we explored some of the pitfalls of these meetings. There are particular difficulties associated with pre-birth meetings. Child protection agencies usually want you to make an assessment of the patient's likely parenting skills. However, general adult psychiatrists have no special expertise in assessing parenting skills, and the impact of mental illness is unpredictable. One is often surprised how well people with serious mental illnesses cope with children and, rather less frequently, one is surprised to find that someone who appeared to have relatively minor mental health problems struggles badly. There is a risk that mothers can develop depressive or delusional ideas about their baby, or neglect them, and it is certainly important to monitor for these things, but they can rarely be foreseen (unless they have happened with previous babies). Generally speaking, parenting skills rest on personality factors and lifestyle, and assessment of these in someone with a mental illness is no different than for people with other types of problems. Of course you often have a view about how well someone is likely to cope, but this is based on ordinary perceptions, not specialist expertise. One has to be cautious about mentioning these views, because on the one hand they are no less valid than the views of anyone else who knows the person, but on the other hand, no matter what caveats you offer, your comments can not be divested of the added significance they carry because they come from a psychiatrist.

Owing to the nature of the post-natal period, with its psychosocial and physical stresses, some women inevitably develop a mental health problem for the first time, from the minor and self-limiting to the severe and persistent. Because mothers and babies can reasonably be regarded as especially vulnerable, and because failure to treat post-natal mental health problems promptly can have long-term consequences, it is appropriate to have a low threshold for mental health assessment. This means being prepared to accept referrals from unusual sources. For example, we know of an instance when a CMHT received a telephone call from the local Registrar of Births, expressing concern about a woman who had just attended to register her baby's birth and to obtain a birth certificate. These days parents often choose unusual names for their children, she said, but Satan didn't seem like a very nice name for a girl.

Having a low threshold for assessment does not imply that there should be a low threshold for treatment, antidepressants and so on. Low-key social interventions are often effective, whether they be practical help or simply someone to talk to. When the problem is more serious, it is important to make a comprehensive assessment. There is a perception that 'puerperal psychosis' is a hormonal reaction. Taken together with appropriate concern over the child's welfare, this can make professionals forget that other contextual factors are just as important in puerperal mental illnesses as in other situations. Neglecting them is bound to result in poor quality treatment plans.

There has long been an awareness that separation of mother and baby in the perinatal period can have a serious impact on bonding and attachment. This in turn can affect the child's development. These are serious matters, and when we started training in psychiatry there were mother and baby units that aimed to keep mother and child together when it was necessary to admit the mother. Most of these have closed, but efforts are still made to admit babies with their mothers to general psychiatric wards, sometimes in distant private sector facilities. Having been involved in a range of such scenarios, we have to say that, in our experience, the arrangement is misguided and counter-productive.

If a mother is able to care for her baby, she usually does not need inpatient care. If she is struggling with this and the baby is brought into hospital, the nursing staff invariably take over the care of the child. Bonding and attachment problems then develop much in the same way as they would have if they had been separated. However, admitting the pair usually delays discharge, and this is exacerbated if the unit is far from home. The problem is that discharge is not determined solely by the mental state of the mother. There is a strong tendency to wait until her parenting skills are unequivocally 'up to scratch'. It usually takes some time to demonstrate this. On the other hand, the mother can be admitted alone and arrangements can be made for the care of the baby at home. Such arrangements can be continued after discharge, which means that the mother can go home as soon as she is well enough, and develop her skills and bonding at her own pace in her own environment. Naturally, such arrangements have to include contact with the baby whilst the mother is in hospital, and due attention has to be given to the baby's care and safety. Generally speaking the usual ways of treating serious mental illnesses work best, and attachment issues are best dealt with by getting the mother better as quickly as possible.

Finally, you are often asked 'Is it all going to happen again the next time I get pregnant?' and, unless it has happened twice, the only truthful answer is that you do not know, but that it is best to assume that it might.

Late disclosure of painful secrets

The last type of complicating factor that we want to explore is the situation where a patient already in treatment makes a disclosure of a significant and painful secret. This can be very difficult to deal with appropriately, and it can completely derail treatment plans. There is, of course, an infinite range of such secrets, which in our personal experience has included confessions to involvement in homicide. However, in routine practice the most common disclosures concern childhood sexual abuse or an eating disorder.

Childhood sexual abuse is a subject that evokes strong emotions, and attitudes to it have caused some deep fissures in the mental health professions, as is illustrated by past controversies over recovered memories, satanic ritual abuse and Freud's theories of infantile sexuality. Childhood sexual abuse is certainly quite common, and it is far from clear why it causes some victims major problems into adulthood, whilst others make a better adjustment to what has happened to them. One suspects that, in many cases, the circumstances in childhood that allowed the abuse to occur are just as damaging as the abuse itself. Exactly the same appears to be true of other bad things that can happen to children, such as bereavement or exposure to persistent bullying.

We have commented elsewhere on a prevalent social attitude that suggests that emotional distress necessarily can and should be resolved through counselling or psychotherapy. This can make the suggestion that it is sometimes best to leave well alone seem callous or dismissive. However, traumatic experiences cannot be eradicated from people's life histories, and the test of whether there should be an intervention rests on the quality of the adjustment that the person has made. The assumption that a history of childhood abuse automatically creates a need for psychological intervention is wrong, because inappropriate intervention can unravel the person's adjustment and leave them feeling more, not less, troubled. Sometimes people complain that counselling about sexual abuse drives them back into the experience in a way that is counter-productive.

Of course, we are not advocating the opposite position either, that intervention is never indicated. The problem lies in helping the person to decide whether a specific intervention is a good idea or not.

It is important to note that we are concerned here with *late* disclosures of childhood sexual abuse, after treatment has commenced. Provided there has been a competent assessment, this means that patients have chosen not to make the disclosure earlier, often in the face of a direct question. They mention it later because they come to trust you, or because someone close to them presses them to, or for a number of other reasons. Nearly always, they feel pretty uncomfortable about making the disclosure, which means that they rarely want (or are ready for) immediate work on the issue. Although such histories are invariably significant contextual or background factors that contribute to the understanding of the person's problems, their relationship to present difficulties may be somewhat tangential. For example, a middle-aged man may be drinking heavily in order to suppress memories of sexual abuse, and the drinking may make him depressed. Eventual help over the abuse may be entirely the right thing to do. On the other hand his depression may have much more to do with being made redundant from his job, with his drinking escalating in order to cope with increasing feelings of depression. He may wonder if his previously undisclosed history of abuse has anything to do with how he feels, in which case it may not, and intervention may simply be a distraction from the main task (i.e. getting him to stop drinking, treating his depression and helping him to find a new job).

Whether or not there should be a psychological intervention with regard to the abuse is not the only consideration. The timing is important as well. There are some questions as to whether psychotherapy should come after the resolution of other problems, or before, in order to allow other interventions to work. Most importantly, people should be allowed to approach psychological interventions at their own speed, when they feel ready. Such therapies usually cause a fair degree of emotional turmoil before people start to feel better about themselves. It is relevant for them to be aware of this in coming to a decision as to timing.

There is a twist to this story. The abuser is often still alive and in contact with children. People who hesitate to make a disclosure are often very ambivalent about the abuser or fearful of the impact on the extended family if the facts come out. The mental health professional can be confronted with a really difficult complication. The patient does not want the authorities to be informed. If you go ahead and do so, they will feel betrayed and they are likely to withdraw from treatment (which may be for a serious illness). They will sometimes say that, if they are questioned by the authorities, they will deny everything, in which case there is a real risk that the patient will not get treated and children will not be protected. Nonetheless, the mental health professional has little option but to inform the authorities anyway. It is usually necessary to take some time (i.e. several interviews) to work on the whole question with the patient, but unfortunately this has to include an acknowledgement that the consequences they fear may come about and there may be insufficient evidence for the authorities to do anything.

Late disclosure of an eating disorder creates some of the same problems, but fortunately it is not as difficult. Some women suffer from eating disorders during adolescence and, whether through treatment or without, settle into a state of chronic stable anorexia nervosa in adult life. They tend to be thin, but not painfully so, but they are often trapped in an intense preoccupation and ritualisation with regard to food and weight. They tend to have very poor self-esteem and to be chronically unhappy. The degree to which they manage to get on with their lives varies considerably, but many pursue careers, get married and have children despite the problem.

Women like this do present for treatment of anorexia nervosa, and some do well despite the poor prognosis of chronic eating disorders. However, some disclose their eating disorder in the course of treatment for a different disorder. The clinician usually feels quite embarrassed under these circumstances at having failed to recognise the significance of their thinness, but in fact a proportion of these women dissemble when you probe about eating problems, only to make a disclosure later. The parallel with childhood sexual abuse lies in the process of making a decision as to whether to do any thing about it or not, and if so, when. One of the potential adverse outcomes of attempts to treat chronic stable anorexia nervosa is to turn it into unstable acute anorexia nervosa (often because people panic at the prospect of weight gain and return to more extreme ways of coping with this). On the other hand, it can be impossible to overcome anxiety and depression without tackling the eating disorder. As before, this is about helping the woman to make a choice rather than forcing her down any particular path.

Conclusion

We have not addressed the full range of complications that can arise in clinical practice here, nor could we. We have tried to draw out some principles, many of which involve striking a balance between ignoring the complication and becoming preoccupied with it. Retaining an organised approach to the adjustment of treatment objectives and treatment planning offers some protection against both of these risks. Above all, we believe that complications can normally be managed within ordinary teams and that the greatest risk to these patients is that they come to be regarded as pariahs or special patients. They cannot be served well when there are disputes over who they 'belong to', nor if they are dealt with in special ways that undermine fundamental and sound principles of mental health practice.

Main points in this chapter

1. Mental health problems do not exist in 'pure culture', and all mental health profes sionals have to be able to manage complicating factors.
2. Substance misuse, and some other volitional behaviours, commonly complicate the treatment of mental illness. It is better to talk with patients in order to try and under- stand the perceived benefits of substance misuse than it is to try to browbeat them into abstinence.
3. The vulnerability and the needs of foetuses and babies have to be taken into account. Overall, mother and baby do best if the mother returns to good mental health and a normal life as quickly as possible, even if this involves a period of separation.

4. The puerperium is a stressful time, and its effect on women's mental health is best understood in the light of this.
5. Painful secrets may demand a specific response, but sometimes it is best to leave well alone.
6. Problems relating to complicating factors can be minimised if one retains an awareness of treatment objectives and attends to treatment planning.

15 Managing risk

The management of risk is not an isolated task. It is an intrinsic part of the work of mental health professionals, and it runs as a continuous theme through all aspects of practice. It involves complexities and ambiguities, and it nearly always involves balancing one type of risk against another (for example, the greater safety achieved by admitting someone to hospital may cause significant long-term problems in other aspects of their life).

Mental health professionals frequently cite risk management as the aspect of their work that causes them greatest anxiety. Risk management was once a matter of professional duty, but this has given way to a more personal type of accountability, whether through litigation or through adverse incident investigations. It is very hard to judge how effective individual practitioners are at identifying and managing risk, because serious incidents occur infrequently. You never know if you have prevented an adverse event. We know from personal experience that, when something bad does happen, defensiveness and guilt cloud your judgement as to whether you could or should have done something differently. Western societies have become markedly intolerant of risk, but no system of care could ever eliminate it. This means that conscientious practitioners will sometimes find themselves criticised or penalised because treatment plans have gone awry. We all have to live with this.

These circumstances create two major pitfalls for mental health professionals. The first is to become complacent ('other people have disasters', 'it won't happen to me', 'it'll probably be alright') or helpless ('if they really want to do it, there's nothing I can do to stop them', 'I can't be responsible for other people's behaviour'). These ways of thinking tend to lead you to inaction over risk (albeit often accompanied by copious documentation lest the worst comes to the worst). This heightens danger, as bad things can happen in anybody's practice, and there is usually something you can do to reduce risk. The second pitfall is overcautious, risk-averse practice, which is usually ineffective, creates problems for patients (as it tends to rely on lengthy admissions and overzealous treatment) and problems for the rest of the service, as resources are diverted in order to control the clinician's anxiety. Somehow, one has to find a path that avoids these pitfalls most of the time.

We have written elsewhere about the first principles of risk assessment (Poole & Higgo, 2006). We will not reiterate them here, as they will be familiar to readers of this book. Suffice to say that they concern careful history taking, identification of known risk factors and an appreciation of the trajectory of the overall situation, all of which has to be tempered by an awareness of the limitations of prediction.

The UK now has an extensive literature of independent inquiry reports concerning homicides carried out by people suffering from mental illness. This appears to demonstrate quite clearly that such events are hard to predict. However, failure to adhere to the first principles of mental health practice is often identified as a major contributory factor (Monro & Rumgay, 2000). This can involve a failure to collate a full history, to understand and communicate the implications of that history, or a failure to assertively follow-up patients who are evasive or aggressive. Our own experience as investigators of untoward incidents strongly suggests that this is true across the full range of serious adverse events. We have also noticed that one particular principle is often broken in the run up to a serious incident, in that an obvious risk indicator is ignored. For example, the patient does or says things that suggest that he is developing ideas of harming someone, but this is dismissed because the clinician's rapport with the patient makes it difficult to accept that a dangerous situation is developing. This is a particular risk when the clinician is working in relative isolation.

The main focus of risk management by mental health services is on dangers that are short term and arise as a direct consequence of mental state abnormalities. For example, when seriously depressed people develop strong suicidal intentions, they usually resolve and disappear when the depression is treated. Mental health services take responsibility for maintaining the patient's safety until the illness, and therefore the danger, has passed. The situation is similar when people become transiently reckless, aggressive or disinhibited as a result of a schizophreniform or manic illness. Although this sounds straightforward, common experience indicates that it rarely is. These situations involve a fine judgement as to the threshold for mental health services to take over responsibility for the person's safety. There is a still more difficult judgement to be made when the patient's mental state is improving, because at some point one has to hand responsibility back to them. Identifying the optimum moment and method of doing this is not easy.

However difficult these situations may be, they involve issues that are dealt with in basic professional training and that tend to be well understood by mental health practitioners. We do not believe that there is a need to dwell upon them here. In this chapter we want to explore two specific and common clinical problems involving difficulties in risk management. These are acute behavioural disturbance and chronic suicidality. They play upon the themes of this book because there are complexities and ambiguities that demand understanding and planning.

Acute behavioural disturbance

When people suffer from mental illness, their behaviour is invariably affected. They may show obvious signs of distress, withdraw from their normal activities or behave in ways that others find bizarre. Acute behavioural disturbance involves more than this. It arises when someone who is suffering from a mental disorder is either behaving in a way that is harmful to themselves or somebody else, or is displaying behaviour that creates an apprehension in those around them that such harm is about to occur. It is different from (and requires a different response to) chronic and habitually disturbed behaviour, in that the situation is changing; the behaviour of concern has arisen de novo or is escalating. It is also different from bad behaviour, which is mostly habitual and personality based (and which is sometimes responsive to peer pressure within an empowered patient group).

Acute behavioural disturbance can be an intrinsic element of a mental state abnormality. Delirium can make otherwise placid people angry or fearful without external provocation, and they can lash out violently. This occurs in people of all ages when they are suffering from acute physical illness. When alcohol withdrawal causes delirium tremens, aggressive and disturbed behaviour can develop with little or no warning. Alcohol intoxication is notoriously potent in releasing aggression. However, in general adult psychiatric practice, these situations of intrinsic disturbance or aggression are relatively uncommon. More frequently, acute behavioural disturbance arises because of the interaction between the mental state abnormality, the environment, and the person's emotional reaction to the situation as he perceives it. Disturbed behaviour is a result of the total situation. It is not a psychopathology embedded in a mental abnormality. This has implications for management, because there is more to be taken into account than drug treatment of mental state abnormalities. Measures relating to the environment and the person's emotional state can make a big difference.

It follows that the things that professionals do can make things worse rather than better, even when their actions are sensible and well intentioned. This is illustrated by the vignette in Box 15.1.

Clearly, in the case described, there were things that the professionals could have done to reduce the risk that the patient would become disturbed as a result of their actions. For example, they could have waited until they had backup before they told Matt that he had to go to hospital. This would have avoided a lengthy build-up of fear and would have reduced the risk of aggression. However, the real point of the vignette is that acute disturbance is an emergent phenomenon. The hospital setting, with its intrinsic emphasis on controlling people, can provoke aggression that would not otherwise arise. This is one good reason for treating people who are acutely unwell at home whenever this is possible. Having said this, acute disturbance in the community can also emerge out of situational factors. It can occur, for example, when people who have been behaving in an odd way for a long time happen to do so in the view of a police officer. In their role of custodians of public order, the police are obliged to do something. Most of us get anxious in the face of the attentions of uniformed police, no matter how kindly their manner. For people who are suffering from psychosis this can provoke aggression. Mental health professionals commonly believe that the number of patients presenting to the service with mania increases during hot weather. We have often wondered if this is because fine weather encourages people to display abnormal behaviour in the open air, where it is noticed, rather than being due to any alteration in the incidence of the disorder.

Of course, once someone is showing acute behavioural disturbance in hospital, it is impossible to discharge them in the hope that they might be less disturbed in the community, because the uncertainties of this course of action represent an unacceptable risk. Acute behavioural disturbance has to be managed promptly and decisively.

Box 15.1 Emergent acute behavioural disturbance

Matt first became unwell at the age of twenty-five. He had a job as a joiner, and was living with his girlfriend when his keen interest in cricket became a worry to him. He noticed that decisions about team selection seemed to be caused by strange ideas that came to him. Over time this developed into a fear that his thinking was having a dangerous effect on the world. He left his job and his partner, and returned to live with his parents. An interview with his GP led to the involvement of the local mental health service, and he spent a few weeks in hospital. He returned to his parents' home feeling calmer, but soon withdrew from follow-up and stopped treatment.

Over the next decade he led a solitary and mostly nocturnal existence. His parents heard him moving around in his room, talking in an animated way, but by day he slept and he spoke little. They pressured him to lead a more normal life, but he would just retreat to his room. One morning he told his parents that he knew that he had to spend the rest of his life in isolation, to prevent his influence causing natural disasters. They felt that something had to be done to rescue him from his hermit existence. On re-assessment, he would not talk to members of the CMHT, and the only options were to either leave him untreated or to admit him to hospital under compulsion. Neither parents nor professionals could see any alternative to admission.

Matt had no history of aggression, and it seemed best to take a low-key approach. Two doctors and a social worker visited to make a formal assessment under the Mental Health Act and, under duress, Matt did speak to them. At the end of the interview he was told by the social worker that he was now legally obliged to come to the hospital. He politely declined, explaining that this would bring catastrophe on anyone who met him, and that it was best that he stayed at home. The social worker then explained that they would, if necessary, return with an ambulance and the police. Matt suddenly became very anxious, and, feeling trapped, assaulted the social worker. The professionals beat a hasty retreat, returning a few hours later with back up as threatened. In the light of the assault, the police went into the house first. Matt became very agitated and lashed out indiscriminately. He was manhandled into a police car and taken to hospital, where he remained highly agitated and fearful. He was nursed on a locked ward, which did nothing to allay his fears. His behaviour remained disturbed for a fortnight, and, as he refused treatment, he had forced intramuscular injections on a number of occasions. Well-intentioned efforts to improve his life had provoked acute behavioural disturbance and a horrible experience for all concerned.

However, whilst hospital management of acute disturbance is a common problem, it is the most hazardous of all psychiatric treatments. The patient is at risk of harming himself and others, but clinicians are also at risk of harming the patient. Patients can die if this type of treatment is not carried out properly (Norfolk, Suffolk and Cambridgeshire Strategic Health Authority, 2003).

The principles of managing acute behavioural disturbance in hospital

The first principle of the safe management of acute disturbance is to recognise that it is bound to happen from time to time. It is therefore important to anticipate it, rather than simply to react when it occurs. The physical environment is important. Small, claustrophobic, overcrowded wards experience more disturbance than wards where there is space, natural light, enclosed external areas and a facility to nurse patients away from too much stimulation. Well-staffed wards allow patients more individual attention, and engagement in activities and human contact can avoid the frustration and fearfulness that drives much of the aggression that is seen in hospital.

Psychiatrists and nurses who are frightened by acute behavioural disturbance make poor decisions. Everyone who is likely to encounter disturbance needs regular training in breakaway techniques, and those staff members who may have to manhandle patients need proper and ongoing training in safe control and restraint techniques. Before these were developed it was common for restraint episodes to degenerate into a general melee. Patients could be asphyxiated by inappropriate control techniques, and stories of staff members being injected instead of the patient are not urban legends. We have seen this happen.

Cardiopulmonary resuscitation is more successful when it is carried out by staff who do it regularly. The same appears to be true of the management of acute disturbance. Staff on wards where acute disturbance is less common may have to pay more attention to remaining prepared for it. Individuals need to understand their roles, and there must be clarity over who is in charge. Ambiguities over authority and decision making processes can cause severe problems when prompt decisions and consistency are needed. However, even when the team and environmental issues are attended to, circumstances can arise that undermine ideal working, for example, during staff sickness or redecoration of wards. If you have to make decisions, you cannot allow yourself to be driven by fearfulness and you must not ask other staff members to do things that they are too frightened to do well.

Patients do not become angry for no reason. The most common causes of anger are fear and frustration. People who have shown disturbed behaviour during previous admissions are likely to show it again. This tends to hold true even when the gap between episodes is measured in decades. It is often possible to anticipate that an individual patient will become acutely disturbed if one takes the trouble to understand the experience of admission from the patient's point of view, and through access to a good history and old records. This may allow you make a plan to avoid disturbed behaviour in the first place or to deal with it before it becomes severe.

The second principle is to be clear and firm with the patient about your concerns and the reasons for your actions. Many patients feel trapped in hospital. Whilst they may not welcome the news that they are likely to be in hospital for weeks, it helps if they can understand what is likely to happen next, and the changes that you are looking for to allow less restrictive treatment. You can only do this if you plan ahead. A time horizon of hours is of little use, because the management of acute disturbance stretches across a time scale of days and sometimes weeks. Plans need to be clearly recorded and must be accessible to everyone who has a role in caring for the patient over the whole twenty-four-hour cycle.

Being firm and clear over that which is non-negotiable is different from being rigid or intimidating. One should be prepared to offer patients choices over matters that do not have an immediate bearing on safety or prompt improvement in their mental state. Giving in to threats is a mistake in life and a bigger mistake in managing acute disturbance, because when you do this, no one is in charge of the situation any more.

Confrontation is not the first choice of approach. Skilful de-escalation and calmness have an important role in managing acute disturbance, but they do not always work. Planning can lead to the recognition that patients are bound to become acutely disturbed. Under these circumstances, it can be a mistake to leave patients unmedicated because of reluctance to manhandle them. Forcible injection of psychotropic medication is a very unpleasant thing to do to someone. It is intrinsically frightening, humiliating and traumatic. It should not be carried out lightly. However, if it is inevitable, then it is better done early, at a time when it can be conducted calmly and with some dignity, than it is to wait for an aggressive episode and to do it reactively. Sometimes, one can involve staff who are particularly trusted by the patient (for example, community staff or inpatient staff who have formed a good relationship in previous admissions), in which case the combination of determination and a friendly face can persuade the patient to accept treatment without a struggle.

The third principle of safe management of these situations is that medication should be used carefully and in the context of an overall plan. The degree of behavioural disturbance does not have an algebraic relationship with the dose of medication that is likely to be needed to calm the patient. Indeed, modern drug regimes involve far lower doses than those used twenty-five years ago, and yet they work much better. Recommendations on exact drug regimes vary over time, but the mainstay of drug treatment of acute disturbance in the context of psychosis is the use of a benzodiazepine with an antipsychotic, both in standard doses. The rationale is that the antipsychotic treats the underlying psychosis whilst the benzodiazepine calms the patient. When an older drug, such as haloperidol, is used it is best to give an antimuscarinic as well, as dystonic reactions are common and do little to persuade the patient of your benign intentions. If intramuscular injection is unavoidable, the use of a medium-acting preparation, such as fluclopenthixol as Clopixol Acuphase, can avoid multiple forced injections and hence reduce the need for repeated confrontation.

When a drug regime is started on admission, or when a regime is altered because the existing regime is failing, it is critical to take into account medications that have already been taken and the impact of drugs and alcohol. There is a need for a clear record of the total medication taken over the previous twenty-four hours, which means avoiding 'PRN' ('as necessary') regimes. The effects of regularly administered medications are far easier to evaluate. If PRN medication is a part of the regime it should be limited to one psychotropic drug, to avoid unpredictable interactions. Patients can go from being agitated and aggressive to being stuporose with alarming speed when complicated combinations of drugs are used. PRN medications that are administered frequently should be made part of a regular regime.

Antipsychotic medication can cause ECG changes, and cardiac arrhythmia is a danger with high dose regimes, which is an excellent reason for avoiding them. A more immediate risk is respiratory depression. Patients who have recently taken opiates or alcohol have unpredictable responses to sedative drugs, especially benzodiazepines. Prescribed methadone is a particular problem because it is long acting. Patients who have recently taken alcohol may have significant quantities in their stomach, and may become more drunk after medication has been administered. Cautious prescribing may not prevent the patient from becoming unconscious, and of course all disturbed patients eventually sleep. Although there is a natural tendency to breath a sigh of relief, this represents a point of significant risk, because the patient can now quietly stop breathing or aspirate vomit. Disturbed people who are not awake need close monitoring, and although there is a reluctance to wake them up, they need to be placed in the recovery position. Above all, nursing staff have to be aware that heavy snoring is a sign of respiratory distress, not of sound sleep.

The initial drug treatment plan needs to include a step-down regime that can be introduced as soon as the acute disturbance passes, in order to avoid continued over-medication. This does not obviate the need for daily medical review, which should normally involve an experienced doctor. Patients who have settled need debriefing, which means an explanation of what has been done to them and why, and an acknowl-edgement that the experience is unpleasant. This maximises the chance of establishing (or re-establishing) a more productive therapeutic relationship later on.

Acute disturbance that does not settle

The most difficult aspect of managing acute disturbance occurs when treatment fails to improve matters. There is a danger of repeated changes of treatment, escalating doses of drugs and incoherent management. As treatment can fail in many different ways, resolving the situation safely can demand both systematic thought and a degree of creativity (see Chapter 14). The main points to bear in mind are:

- *Are we being too impatient?* Disturbed behaviour can take days or weeks to settle, and sometimes all you can do is contain the behaviour until the person gets better. Repeated changes of medication can slow improvement rather than hastening it.
- *Is treatment making things worse?* Patients who are delirious may deteriorate when they are given benzodiazepines (which are best avoided in confused patients). Older antipsychotic medications, such as chlorpromazine, have a role in managing acute disturbance, but only in lower doses. At high doses they have toxic antimuscarinic effects, which can drive excitement.
- *Is the diagnosis right?* When patients are very disturbed it can be difficult to tell what is really wrong with them. Sometimes a patient who was thought to be psychotic is found to be delirious when re-examined in the light of a failure to improve. The management of the two situations is different. Occasionally the psychiatric diagnosis

is right but there is a complicating factor, such as a physical illness, that is causing or exacerbating disturbed behaviour.

- *Could covert drug misuse be complicating things?* Psychiatric inpatient units, in common with all other institutions in the UK, have a black market in cannabis. Cannabis can make people intermittently very irritable. In our experience, continuous disturbed behaviour is rarely attributable to drug use. The drugs most likely to cause disturbance lasting days are large doses of amphetamine or, rarely, MDMA (ecstasy). There is also a black market in alcohol, which is a potent cause of unexpected aggression, but it too is rarely a cause of continuous problems.
- *Is overstimulation contributing?* Two or more disturbed patients can create a buzzing emotional tension on a ward, which can then prevent both of them from improving. Similarly, some kinds of visitors can inadvertently be unhelpfully emotionally stimulating, though controlling this is difficult, as visitors are important to patients.
- *Are some members of the staff failing to adhere to the plan?* This happens. It is hardly surprising that it renders treatment less effective. It can have a number of different origins, including disagreement with the plan, being intimidated by the patient and incompetence. It is, in its nature, covert. It is usually detected through careful reading of drug administration charts and contemporaneous nursing notes (which in any case is always a good thing to do).

Twenty-five years ago, sodium amytal and paraldehyde were occasionally used when all else failed. The result of amytal could be that the patient developed pneumonia. Paraldehyde is safe, but it makes the patient smell, and injections cause an inflammatory reaction. We cannot say that these drugs have no role, but if they do, it is only in extremis. If one is struggling so badly that dangerous or unpleasant drugs seem necessary, it is time to seek advice. Some units call upon the police to restore order when treatment fails. The police are ill equipped for the task. If you involve them in inpatient treatment, they cannot function well. In our experience, they tend to have a low threshold for the use of seriously unhelpful measures, such as tear gas and stun guns.

Chronic suicidality

Chronic suicidality is a risk management problem that is in many ways the converse of acute behavioural disturbance, because it involves very long-term factors and cannot be resolved by trying to control the patient. The number of people who are chronically suicidal is small, but there are one or two such patients amongst most general adult psychiatrists' caseload. They are highly anxiety provoking, and management of the situation often involves choosing between equally unsatisfactory alternatives.

We are not referring here to people who repeatedly lacerate themselves. This is a tension relief strategy, and seldom involves a wish to die. Nor are we concerned here with that larger group of people who repeatedly take overdoses in order to influence the behaviour of other people. People who are chronically suicidal are usually ambivalent about their own death, both fearing and welcoming the prospect. This may be due to very difficult feelings, such as self-loathing, that are painful and unremitting. Death offers the prospect of non-existence and hence relief. Sometimes people feel that their lives are irredeemably meaningless and burdensome, because they have no satisfactory relationships and can see no way forward (people with chronic or terminal physical disease can arrive at a similar conclusion). A substantial proportion are chronically angry with those who have abused them or let them down. They have aggressive suicidal feelings, in the belief that taking their own lives will cause pain and remorse in others. There are other antecedents, but chronic suicidality almost invariably arises out of the interaction between deep-seated personality characteristics and life trajectory.

People who are chronically suicidal do not belong to a separate diagnostic category. The factors that generate continuous suicidal feelings intertwine with vulnerability to a variety of mental illnesses. Chronic suicidality can arise in the absence of mental illness, but many people who have a fixed suicidal intention do suffer from recurrent episodes of illness. They are not suicidal throughout their lives. What marks them out is that once they have developed suicidal urges, the feelings do not go away even when their mental health improves. Box 15.2 sets out one such unhappy life history.

There are a number of factors that cause major problems for clinicians when they are trying to help people who hold long-term suicidal plans:

- Mental health professionals cannot ignore suicide risk. They have an ethical and legal obligation to strive to preserve life. However, the risk is long term and unlikely to alter quickly. Over time, the immediate risk varies with circumstances. The clinician has to make judgements that are highly subjective, and which are therefore easy to get wrong. This tends to make professionals anxious in dealing with people with these problems, and clinician anxiety does little to assist clear thinking.
- The patient and the clinician have a clash in their agendas which cannot be resolved. This makes it difficult (though not impossible) to establish a positive therapeutic relationship with truly shared objectives.
- Many patients with long-term suicidal ideas resist doing things to improve their situation on the rationale that it is pointless because they will soon be dead. Clinicians inevitably experience this as patients' refusal to take responsibility for their own well being or, to put it another way, as a serious motivational problem. It is always frustrating to work with people with poor motivation to change, and this can turn into anger and hostility towards the patient.
- If someone has been determined for a long time to kill himself, it is not difficult for him to succeed, even in the face of strenuous efforts by mental health services to prevent this. This can make clinicians feel helpless and that failure is unavoidable.

The combination of anxiety, hostility and helplessness in a clinician who is likely to be called to account if the patient does kill himself is toxic. It invites the clinician to either reject the patient on the grounds that nothing can be done (which is not necessarily true) or to become highly controlling (which does nothing to help the patient to take responsibility for his own well being and sometimes crystallises suicidal plans as the ultimate expression of autonomy). The forces driving the clinician towards these pitfalls are powerful. Most of us are likely to have the experience from time to time of finding ourselves trapped in a situation where we knowingly fall into one or other of these

Box 15.2 A spiral of loss

Roger was an intelligent child. His father was a long-distance lorry driver, and a heavy drinker who was violent to his wife and children. Roger liked primary school because it was orderly and predictable, and he found haven in the local library, where he developed a love of reading. His father despised Roger's studiousness, and teased him mercilessly about his lack of sporting ability.

Roger secured a place at grammar school, but he was bullied and left without taking his final exams. He found work as a warehouseman, and met a girl at the library. She was several years older than him, and had two children by a previous partner. She shared his interest in books and literature, and they married when Roger was nineteen. He soon came to realise that his wife had a serious drinking problem. Unable to influence her, he started drinking with her. The couple had three children in the first five years of the marriage. Life in the household was difficult. They were overcrowded, the children were demanding, and the couple struggled with the upkeep of the house and the bills. They still read voraciously and often drunkenly argued about the merits of the books they read. They had a particularly violent fight that was provoked by a disagreement as to whether Charles Dickens was a genius or an incontinent sentimentalist. Roger started going to the library to avoid the atmosphere at home.

One evening, when Roger was at the library, his wife ran out of wine. She told her nine-year-old daughter that she was to look after the other children, and she set off for the off-licence. She had done this many times before, but on this occasion she bumped into a friend, who persuaded her to go to the pub for a quick drink. Meanwhile at home, the couple's two-year-old fell and hit her head. There was a small cut on her scalp which bled copiously, frightening the nine-year-old, who went to the neighbours for help. Realising that five children were unattended, they called social services. Roger returned from the library to find his wife absent and social workers putting the children into cars to convey them to foster care.

Roger and a social worker were still awake when his wife returned at breakfast time, drunk. On learning what had happened, she blamed Roger, and there was a ferocious argument. In the weeks that followed, the child protection agencies made efforts to return the children to their parents, but the couple were now drinking and arguing more than ever. The children were permanently placed in care. Roger's wife left him for a man she met at the pub. Alone in the house he drank and read, but he made sure he was sober when he visited his children. He lost his job for being drunk at work, and six months later his mother died from a heart attack. Roger's finances were perilous, and he moved in with his father because it was cheaper than living alone. His father's disdain was sharpened by accusations that Roger had never been a real man, he could not hold a job and he could not control his wife. By now Roger was seriously depressed, and one evening he tried to hang himself from his bedroom door. He was saved when his father investigated the banging of Roger's feet against the door.

Roger was admitted to a psychiatric unit, where he was detoxified and treated with antidepressants. After some weeks his mood lifted, and he willingly participated in the therapeutic activities that were arranged for him in the community. However, when asked, he told the staff that he had nothing to live for, that he had failed in everything, and that, whilst he was grateful for their help, he would rather be dead. Within a few months he was back to an isolated life of reading and drinking, with only his critical and hostile father for company. Roger stopped visiting his children in order to protect them from the trauma of his planned suicide.

Over the next few years there were two further suicide attempts, the first a serious overdose and the second an attempt to jump in front of a train. He was admitted to hospital, and on each occasion his mental state improved, but his long-term suicidal plans did not alter. Eventually he was visited at home by his eldest daughter, who had reached the age of eighteen. She was shocked at his deteriorated condition. She accused him of having neglected his children from the outset, and told him that he would never see her again. A week later he took another major overdose that required treatment in an intensive care unit. Once he was medically fit, he was transferred back to the psychiatric unit. After two days the staff had to break bad news. His father had been crossing the road on the way to visit him when he was hit by a car and killed. Roger had always been a quiet and compliant patient, but now he became very agitated. There was nothing and no one left. He wanted to discharge himself so that he could go to the town centre and throw himself off the car park roof. The staff had no option but to detain him under the Mental Health Act.

This time his depression did not respond to treatment. He was mainly silent and kept himself away from staff and patients. He would reluctantly tell the nurses that he had reached the absolute bottom, total failure, certified insane and useless. The psychiatrist wanted him to have ECT, to which he agreed. That evening Roger slipped out of the ward when visitors were leaving, bought and consumed a bottle of whisky and threw himself in front of a train. When the ambulance arrived, he was dead.

positions, unable to avoid it because there is no alternative course available to us. This is an unpleasant and unhelpful experience for all concerned.

There are some ways of thinking about these situations that sometimes help in finding a more constructive way forward. They are not rules, and cannot be applied indiscriminately, because they involve therapeutic risk taking. The willingness to take calculated risks in pursuit of a therapeutic objective is an essential characteristic of all good clinicians. However, the appropriateness of risk taking is embedded in the overall situation, because the size and nature of the risk has to be balanced against the likelihood and degree of therapeutic benefit. Taking a huge risk in pursuit of an implausible goal is not therapeutic risk taking, it is recklessness. Furthermore, in taking risks, one has to be mindful of the alternatives, and the likelihood that these might be more productive. It is easier to justify risk taking when alternative strategies are unlikely to achieve very much.

- *Sharing your thinking with the patient.* Clinicians tend to be reluctant to share their worries about patients with them, but if you do, it can work surprisingly well. This is especially true where there is a clash of agendas over risk. 'I understand that you see taking your life as the solution, but I think there may be another way forward, and my job is to try to persuade you that this is true' is a position that can be effective in engaging the ambivalence that is usually a marked feature of chronic suicidality. Most people want hope, and many are willing to pursue a different strategy whilst holding the default position that they will take their life if it fails.

- *Acknowledgement that suicide is an option.* 'I know you intend to kill yourself and I'm going to stop you' is not a constructive position because it makes you part of the suicidal nexus. This is likely to be the position of other people close to the patient, and, in recapitulating it, you are at risk of simply becoming part of the problem. The acknowledgement that you cannot ultimately prevent the person from taking his life has the advantage of placing you outside of this nexus. The statement is also true, and it can free the therapeutic relationship from unhelpful and ineffective issues of control. The acknowledgement has to be conducted with considerable care, because it is dangerous to convey the impression that you either do not care if the patient kills himself or that you are somehow condoning it.

- *Awareness of factors that heighten short-term risk.* There are usually factors in a given situation that are likely to change a long-term plan into an immediate intention. Episodes of frank depression, heavy drinking, losses and rejections are examples. The secret to success in some of these situations is the combination of toleration of long-term risk but prompt intervention when predictably more dangerous events occur.

- *Recognition that suicidal plans are only likely to be abandoned if the person's life situation improves.* There is rarely much chance that a simple intervention will alter long-term plans of suicide. Long-term suicidal thinking is only likely to change if the person's life changes in a significant way. This demands attention to the patient's daily activities and lifestyle.

- *Avoidance of pressure to relinquish suicidal plans.* If you create an expectation that patients will disavow their plans in the short term, they will sometimes oblige. This may relieve your anxiety, but it is rarely sincere. The patients are generally either trying to please you or trying to avoid you thwarting them. When intervention is successful, people will eventually tell you that they have decided that they want to live. This has invariably become evident indirectly much earlier, in the form of optimistic plans and pleasure in new activities. Browbeating people into denying suicidal plans undermines fragile therapeutic relationships.

- *Track the trajectory of the situation.* Once you form a functional therapeutic relation-ship with a chronically suicidal patient, it can be difficult to recognise the trajectory of the total situation. Warm rapport with a patient who evidently values you is bound to give the impression that things are moving in the right direction. This is not nec-essarily true, and the patient's life circumstances can be deteriorating, moving him closer to suicide. The best way of tracking the trajectory is to periodically discuss the case with an experienced colleague, who is likely to be in a better position to recognise the overall direction of travel. These are the cases that most need to be taken to supervision.

- *The utility of hospital admission.* Lengthy hospital admissions tend to be a disaster in the management of chronic suicidality, especially when they involve legal compulsion. At best, long admissions delay suicide, and sometimes they simply lead to death in hospital. They can worsen the patient's life situation and deepen hopelessness. They are incompatible with the formation of a therapeutic alliance with patients holding long-term suicidal plans. Long admissions have no clear end point or achievable objectives, and malignant alienation from inpatient staff is common. Short-term admissions to achieve focussed objectives can be helpful, for example, in order to treat an intercurrent depression or heavy drinking, but even here there is a risk that the intended brief admission turns into an unintended long admission because of the institutional response to someone who continues to express suicidal plans. This means that admissions have to be carefully planned. If possible, it is useful to have clarity from the outset of treatment as to the circumstances which might be constructively dealt with through admission, and those which would not.

- *Defensive measures.* Defensive practice is a bad thing, because it places the clinician's needs above the patient's. However, a degree of defensiveness can be helpful, in so far as it helps to contain the clinician's anxiety. Dealing with long-term suicidality always involves a degree of risk taking, and sometimes things will go wrong and the clinician is called to account through the courts or inquiries. The key defensive measure is to discuss cases with team colleagues and to take care of recording the development of your thinking and the rationale behind plans and decisions. Under most circumstances, you are protected if you can demonstrate from contemporaneous records that you thought things through and made reasonable judgements.

The management of long-term risk has a large number of pitfalls and no invariable pathways forward. Success is by no means impossible, but it is difficult and draining. There are obvious parallels between the management of chronic suicidality and the management of violent people who become more dangerous when they become mentally ill (though there are also significant differences). What makes the practice of psychiatry really interesting, if sometimes very stressful, is the task of making therapeutic progress despite the emotional and intellectual challenges of situations like this.

When the worst happens

It is an unavoidable fact of mental health practice that sometimes the worst will happen. All clinicians eventually have to deal with the aftermath of death and other bad outcomes. In recent years, policy makers and managers of mental health services have recognised that the apportioning of blame can obstruct efforts to learn from adverse incidents, but their efforts to conduct constructive reviews have been impeded by rising professional anxiety over litigation, inquiries and publicity. The big problem with serious untoward incidents is that, far from improving practice through 'learning the lessons', the aftermath can have an adverse effect on clinicians' ability to practise effectively.

In our experience, when a patient takes his own life, the clinician's first reaction is guilt and a loss of self-confidence. Individuals vary considerably in the extent to which this is accompanied by fearfulness for their own professional standing and career prospects. Sometimes, clinicians are so gripped by panic that they try to improve their position by doing something seriously stupid, such as altering the case notes. This type of overly defensive response, when discovered, has far worse consequences for the clinician than the incident itself. Even when people keep their nerve and do not seem to overreact, their practice is temporarily or permanently coloured by caution and strenuous efforts to avoid a recurrence. Needless to say, this does little to reduce risk, and causes a deterioration in the quality of their work. There is a major risk of arbitrary generalisation, whereby all situations that have similarities with the index case are treated as very dangerous. Clinical decisions are no longer made logically but are driven by efforts to undo the previous events or to contain the clinician's phobic anxieties.

The primary reason for holding team reviews after deaths is to avoid this outcome. Although it is sometimes possible to reflect and learn from serious incidents, team reviews are not ideal mechanisms to achieve this. Proper and full reflection is usually only possible after the immediate emotional reaction has passed, when all the facts have been collated. In the aftermath there is a need to support those immediately affected by the death, namely family and friends of the patient. This needs to be timely. It is not always welcomed, but it should be offered.

Teams tend to look inward in times of stress, but there are often other professionals who are outside of the team who have had a close involvement with the patient, for example, in primary care. Immediate clinical reviews should involve all the professionals, whether in the team or not. Reviews like this need an external facilitator, because everyone is likely to be upset, and group processes can run out of control. This kind of debriefing and initial examination of the management of the situation does not confer absolute protection against either distress or inappropriate alterations in professional behaviour, but it certainly helps.

Main points in this chapter

1. Even uncomplicated risk management problems involve difficult judgements, particularly with respect to the threshold and timing for taking responsibility away from the patient and handing it back again.
2. Acute behavioural disturbance is usually a consequence of the total situation, not the patient's mental state alone. Although drug treatment is important, it is not the most significant part of managing disturbed behaviour.
3. Teamwork, anticipation, planning, and explanation to the patient minimise the risk of acute disturbance and of hazardous treatment.
4. Chronic suicidality is difficult to manage and evokes negative feelings in clinicians. Nonetheless, it is possible to help people overcome long-term suicidal plans.

5. Management often involves a combination of therapeutic engagement and risk taking. Efforts to control the patient, particularly through lengthy hospital admissions, should be approached with caution as they can be counter-productive.

6. When there is a serious untoward incident, there is a need for an externally facilitated team debriefing, in order to avoid inappropriate alterations to clinical practice.

Medical training tends to focus on acute episodes of illness and on ways of helping people to overcome them. Mental health training also emphasises this aspect of treatment. Most of the technologies and the greater part of the evidence base in psychiatry are orientated towards the short term. However, the acute illness model is only applicable to a small part of the work of mental health services, and clinicians can find it altogether more difficult to help people to stay well in the long term. Helping people to avoid relapse and to develop self-management strategies calls upon a wide range of skills in areas of clinical endeavour with a sparse evidence base.

The simplest model of mental health intervention involves a clinician doing something of a technical nature with a clear-cut start and finish. The problem is permanently resolved, and there is no need for the person to do anything more about his mental health. This model of illness–intervention–cure is based on the surgical paradigm that dominates acute health services. It exists as an assumed model in the funding arrangements for mental health services in many countries, but it is based on a false premise. Even if one has a strong attachment to a disease model, it is difficult to deny that the relationship between illness and contextual factors is profound. This is just as true of cancer or arthritis as it is of mental disorder. Even where intervention is simple and short term (for example, where a depressed person sees an office-based psychiatrist, is prescribed an antidepressant and gets better), the experience is likely to have changed the way people think about themselves and their lives. Where they remain well, this is likely to rest upon changes that they have made, or which have occurred, in their lives. These may not have been instigated by the clinician; positive change is by no means the exclusive territory of professionals.

Recovery rests on a sense of well being and of personal autonomy. It does not imply invulnerability to the return of symptoms or to relapse. It can mean recognising the circumstances under which symptoms are likely to recur or worsen and having strategies to control these situations. For example, this may mean keeping an ampoule of intramuscular antipsychotic medication in the fridge, to be administered when the need arises. There are many routes to recovery but they all involve the person taking responsibility for their own well being. The clinician's job is to facilitate the development of strategies that work, rather than didactically creating them.

No one enters psychiatric treatment in the expectation that it will be life long. Nonetheless, one of the marked features of state-funded mental health services, such as the UK's, is exactly the fact that many patients stay in follow-up for a very long time. The ability to work with people over long periods, without worrying about funding running out, is a strength of the British system. Some problems do take a considerable time to resolve, and a small proportion of mental illnesses prove to be intractable. However, it is also a weakness of the system. Psychiatrists often lack clarity on the eventual discharge plan, which creates an implicit expectation of indefinite follow-up. Patients come to share this expectation, and this can be destructive. The belief that your well being is forever dependent on seeing a mental health professional is no less damaging than the sense that you are unwillingly caught in a mental health system that offers no route back to freedom.

Although indefinite follow-up is sometimes appropriate, it is not the best route to recovery. Planning for discharge is an important part of the process of moving towards recovery, which means the clinician has to have some faith in the patient's ability to manage their disorder. However, where people have an enduring mental health problem, it is also necessary to ensure that there is a route back to professional help in the event of the unforeseen. If barriers to return are so high that you can only access services when you are very ill, then discharge involves a major gamble. It is unrealistic to expect people to take chances with their health in this way. Recovery is facilitated by the combination of discharge and accessible services. There is a big difference between dependent follow-up and easy access to professional help when you know you need it.

Generally speaking, recovery and staying well are not contingent on technical manoeuvres, such as particular drug treatments, important though these can be. Staying well involves a configuration of personal strategies, of back up services and, most of all, a way of thinking that is shared by clinicians and (ex-)patients. Cycles of relapse are usually driven by contextual factors. Overall, these are more powerful in determining what happens than are intrinsic factors related to the nature of the illness. The clinician's task is often centred on helping people to break destructive cycles and to find new ways of handling problems.

Medication is just one part of a broader strategy to stay well. There are some dilemmas associated with the long-term use of medication.

Long-term medication

Schizophrenia and bipolar affective disorder are both intrinsically long-term disorders with a strong tendency to persistence or recurrence. There are drug treatments that demonstrably make a significant difference when patients are acutely unwell. There are well-established, long-term medication regimes for both conditions. All conscientious clinicians recognise the importance of drug treatments as part of a strategy to stay well when you have these illnesses. However, using these drug treatments successfully is often surprisingly complicated, and there are real ambiguities that are evident both from clinical experience and from the literature.

Schizophrenia and bipolar affective disorder have some similarities, with substantial overlap in presentation and treatment, but there are also major differences between the two disorders. People with schizophrenia have to set the adverse effects of medication against symptom control, finding an optimal balance of the two. People with bipolar affective disorder, on the other hand, can often experience a complete remission of symptoms without medication against the background of a continuing risk of relapse. Both scenarios can occur in both disorders, but, overall, issues of control of continuous symptoms are more common for people suffering from schizophrenia and issues of prevention of relapse are more common for people with bipolar affective disorder.

Bipolar affective disorder

There has been a fierce debate over the usefulness of lithium carbonate in preventing relapse in bipolar affective disorder for quite a long time. The skeptics and enthusiasts have taken polarised positions on the basis of what is essentially undisputed data. Many clinicians with no particular emotional commitment to either side of the controversy recognise that the academic rhetoric reflects their internalised mixed feelings and the uncertainties intrinsic to a common clinical problem (Geddes *et al.*, 2004).

The main relevant facts about lithium are as follows:

- Lithium is an effective anti-manic agent. Its antidepressant properties are far weaker (when used as a monotherapy).
- Continuous treatment with lithium prevents manic relapse at least as effectively as other agents, and it may be more effective than other mood stabilisers.
- Episodes of depression tend to follow episodes of mania in established bipolar affective disorder, though depressions can occur independently. It is not clear whether lithium is a true mood stabiliser or whether its action is largely due to its anti-manic effects, i.e. by preventing manic episodes the subsequent depressive episodes are also avoided.
- No mood stabiliser confers absolute protection against relapse in all patients. They reduce the frequency and severity of relapse for most people.
- Abrupt discontinuation of lithium can provoke a manic episode that would not have occurred otherwise.
- Lithium is potentially toxic stuff, and higher blood levels cause unpleasant side effects such as diuresis, tremor and a metallic taste. Lower levels cause fewer side effects, but are less effective. The requirement for routine blood testing over long periods is tiresome.
- Whether or not they intend to, all patients on lithium have to stop it from time to time, if only because everyone suffers from gastrointestinal upsets occasionally.

This raises a series of questions. Although lithium is technically effective, is this negated in the real world by its tendency to provoke relapse when it is discontinued? If this is true, are there strategies that can avoid the problems associated with lithium? Are other, less technically effective, mood stabilisers to be preferred, because discontinuation does not provoke manic episodes? Is lithium appropriate for some people and not others? How can clinician and patient decide what to do for the best in the face of ambiguous evidence?

The scientific debate on these matters has been important, not least because it has shone a light on a well-recognised clinical problem, but there are no clear answers that can be easily derived from the literature. In practice, some patients find lithium helpful and others do not. As no drug confers absolute protection from relapse, there is always a need to have strategies to deal with the possibility of symptoms re-emerging. The supposition that the drug treatment stands alone, separated from contextual factors, is false. It is not true that people with bipolar affective disorder can simply take the medication and carry on with life as if they have never been ill. Everyone suffers from stresses in everyday life, and everyone has bad times when they feel low. Most people have good times when they feel expansive and on top of the world. Even after years of good mental health it is natural that people who have suffered from bipolar affective disorder should worry that fluctuations in their mood might augur a relapse, and this is a realistic concern. Alcohol binges are not good for anyone, but they may provoke relapse if you suffer from bipolar affective disorder. People with this illness need an awareness of the situations that might destabilise their mental health, an ability to evaluate changes in their mood and strategies to cope with stress. For many people, the decision to use a mood stabiliser, and finding an effective drug that they can tolerate, is necessary but not sufficient to stay well.

Prophylaxis is not always the optimal approach in bipolar affective disorder. Some patients do better with a strategy based on the recognition of early signs of relapse and self-initiated use of an antipsychotic. Under all circumstances, drug treatment has to be a coherent part of an overall strategy to stay well. The drugs can only ever do part of the job.

Schizophrenia

There are some parallels in the long-term management of schizophrenia. For a small group of people, the disorder only manifests itself intermittently. Under these circumstances, an 'early warning signs' and self-initiated medication regime can be appropriate. For most people, schizophrenia is a continuous disorder and symptoms return or worsen quite quickly (though not immediately) on discontinuation of medication. Whilst this makes the task of finding an optimal drug regime more complex, it does not change the principle that staying well involves a broad approach to the management of stressors and maintenance of good mental health. Although intermittent drug regimes do not work well for most people with schizophrenia, control over dosage according to circumstances can be an important component of a self-management strategy. It can help to avoid the adverse consequences of continuous high doses of antipsychotic medication.

Intermittent and variable dose regimes, controlled by the patient, seem to have much to commend them, and in our experience they can work well. However, they are not a panacea, and they have some major drawbacks. The penalty for failure is high, and the evidence base supporting such regimes is limited. Patients have to be warned about this. Whilst some patients like variable regimes, they can only be successful when the patient has a really good understanding of their disorder. Some people with serious mental disorders want a variable dose regime because they do not accept that they have a continuing mental health problem, and choose a flexible regime as a compromise between their own wishes and the wishes of those around them. In our experience, the combination of denial and flexible medication regimes is a bad one, and the approach rarely works under these circumstances.

The dilemma of success

Long-term drug treatment has a further problem, which lies in deciding what to do when it appears to be entirely successful. Nearly everyone taking psychotropic medication aspires to come off it eventually. The prospect of lifelong medication is daunting, even when the medication has no unpleasant side effects. When people with bipolar affective disorder stay well for many years, or when people do well after a first episode of schizophrenia, there is a real dilemma in knowing how best to advise them. There is no proper evidence base for medication discontinuation after prolonged good mental health, and although there is a good deal of accumulated clinical experience of managing the situation in different ways, it is hard to know how to best advise individual patients.

Bipolar affective disorder follows a particularly unpredictable course. Clusters of episodes followed by protracted periods of good mental health are common. There is a lifetime risk of eventual relapse that can be quantified for populations but not for individuals. The classic interpretation of Kraepelin is that he regarded what we now call schizophrenia as a chronic and progressive disorder. However, it is clear that he recognised that this was not invariable. It is evident that clinicians working in mental health services long before the invention of antipsychotic medications knew that some people presenting with full blown schizophreniform episodes would eventually get better, and would sometimes stay well thereafter. For the modern clinician, the problem is that, when someone has been well for a long time on medication, it is impossible to know for certain if this has happened as a result of treatment. It is reasonable to assume that medication has made a difference for the majority of patients, but it is impossible to know what would have happened to individual patients if they had not taken it.

Most experienced clinicians are familiar with the dilemma of conflicting past experience. It is distressing to preside over a situation where a patient has made a good recovery from a serious mental illness, only to experience a full-blown relapse when there is a planned withdrawal of medication. It is also common experience that some people who you think will relapse under these circumstances do not become ill, at least in the short run. These risks cannot be reliably quantified. The best way forward is to share the ambiguities with the patient. When they choose to take their chances on relapse, it is often possible to move from one strategy to another, for example from a fixed medication regime to a variable dose strategy, moving towards discontinuation in a stepwise manner.

Psychosocial interventions

Cognitive behaviour therapy (CBT) is the dominant psychological treatment of our time, and we would not seek to deny its importance. We do doubt whether a mental health culture that places an emphasis on a single treatment approach is really healthy, as CBT has its limitations, and other approaches have some value. CBT-based psychosocial interventions for psychosis have become widely available. They are important tools in helping people to understand and manage their disorder. The fact that they do not abolish symptoms is not necessarily a major limitation. However, we have long been puzzled that CBT-based psychosocial interventions have proven so popular compared with behavioural family therapy aimed at reducing expressed emotion. Evidence for the effectiveness of the latter has been available since the 1970s, and yet it has never really caught on as an essential component of routine treatment.

One suspects that the difficulty with family intervention is the logistical awkwardness of formal family work and the fact that CBT fits better with the individual treatment paradigm that is central to the professional culture of health workers (though not social care workers). The modern evidence suggests that individual and family work are roughly similar in effectiveness. Neither seems to be startlingly effective as a stand-alone treatment (Thornicroft & Susser, 2001; Pilling *et al.*, 2002). However, this is true of most mental health interventions when studied in a research setting. Aggregated research findings on interpersonal therapies can conceal a greater effectiveness for these approaches in the hands of particularly skilled individuals. Departures from manualised programmes to meet the needs of individual families and patients are incompatible with methodological rigour in research but may be important in clinical practice. There is a widespread perception that formal psychosocial interventions have made an important contribution to the management of serious mental illness, and the more modest findings of research do not necessarily contradict this. Family intervention and CBT have had a significant impact on the way that clinicians of all disciplines think about serious mental illness. It seems to us that these ways of thinking inform interventions and treatment planning far beyond the formal use of specific psychosocial technologies. If standard treatment has incorporated ideas from, say, family intervention to good effect, it might be difficult to demonstrate the effectiveness of formal family intervention over standard care. Similar processes have been invoked to explain the lack of demonstrable superiority of psychiatric assertive community treatment over standard care in the UK (Burns *et al.*, 2007).

Psychosocial and family interventions, whether formal or not, may have a significant role in helping people stay well, but, just like prophylactic medication, they are not cure-all, stand-alone interventions. They have to be part of a total approach that aims at improving the patient's repertoire of useful coping strategies, their resilience and hence their well being. Whether or not formalised therapy is part of the package, the arena for co-ordinating and managing the work of facilitating recovery is the therapeutic relationship between the patient and his key clinician. In the British system, this might be a psychiatrist, but it might equally be a care co-ordinator from another discipline. There is a generic problem solving approach to dealing with situational problems and everyday stresses that has come into mental health services from social work. The approach is rarely articulated or studied, though the research on psychiatric assertive community treatment does identify it as a key component of care (Killaspy, 2007). In practice, it is a major element of the work of all CMHTs. In our opinion, it is likely that it is a major factor in helping people to stay well. It certainly has been important in making mental health services more user friendly and in rendering mental health interventions more relevant to people's lives. Whilst the approach has come from social care, it works best if it is part of the repertoire of all mental health disciplines. Psychiatrists' particular expertise arises from their background in biological sciences, but their effectiveness as clinicians is greatly enhanced by an ability to understand and work within the social environment.

Personality factors

Of all the contextual factors that can obstruct recovery, two stand out as particularly potent. The first is daytime television. There is a strong association between extended exposure and a failure to recover from mental illness. Whilst daytime TV is undoubtedly repetitive, mindless and depressing, it seems unlikely that it has a direct anti-therapeutic effect (although its classic accompaniments for young men – a four pack of super-strength lager and a spliff – are more damaging). More likely, people watch a lot of daytime TV because their life lacks activity and meaning. Helping people to find meaningful and satisfying activities is a central task. It may or may not lead to paid employment, but recovery cannot occur in the context of a purposeless existence.

The second obstruction is personality factors. Problems rooted in personality development and frank personality disorder have a high prevalence amongst users of adult mental health services, even where a primary diagnosis of personality disorder is an exclusion criterion (Keown *et al.*, 2002). Some clinicians adopt the position that personality problems have nothing to do with mental health services. This position is sterile and untenable. An ability to work with people who have problems at the personality level is an essential capability for clinicians of all disciplines. This is not to say that all personality problems are amenable to psychiatric intervention or that people with personality problems are necessarily best helped within mental health services. However, if one is aiming to help people to improve their lives and to overcome mental illness, skills in helping them to overcome personality difficulties are essential.

Personality and personality disorder are difficult and complex subjects. There is a range of ways of understanding them, each with some limitations. A broad way of thinking about personality problems that has a basic utility is that some people lack an available adaptive behavioural response to deal with the circumstances they find themselves in. They therefore deploy a response that is within their repertoire, but which is maladaptive in the current circumstances. When that behavioural response fails to resolve problems, they continue to deploy it rather than searching for a new one. This mismatch between circumstances and behaviour can occur in anyone in extreme circumstances. For people who have had pervasively bad childhood experiences, the damage to their personality development can be such that there is a mismatch under quite ordinary circumstances. Personality problems in clinical practice are strung across a spectrum from difficulties experienced by people with essentially normal personality development who are struggling with extreme circumstances to people who are struggling with ordinary problems of daily existence because of damaged personality

Box 16.1 The last roll of the dice

Dr Ashton's first impression of Vince was not promising. Vince was a tense, unsmiling man, who made little eye contact but whose intelligence was exposed by flashes of deadpan humour. Vince was a veteran of psychiatric treatment by five previous psychiatrists over twelve years. 'After my thirtieth birthday,' he told her 'I decided that if life was going to go on like this, I might as well kill myself. I'm going to have one last try at treatment, and if this fails, I'm out of here.'

Vince had attracted a range of diagnoses in the past, including alcohol dependency, paranoid, avoidant and borderline personality disorders, and recurrent depressive illness. He certainly did suffer episodes of severe depression with biological features, but there was also an obvious personality problem. He found it difficult to trust other people, and avoided social contact. He took offence easily. He had little confidence in his own abilities. He drank alcohol in a 'lost weekend' pattern, weeks of abstinence punctuated by several days of continuous intoxication which often ended in his arrest or in an attendance at A&E following an act of self-harm. Treatment with antidepressants had helped in the short term, but had done nothing to alter the pattern of his life. Earlier referrals to a therapeutic community and for psychoanalytic psychotherapy had not been productive, because of Vince's reluctance to engage with other people.

Vince was living a barren life. He had no friends, and his only social contact was with his mother for Sunday lunch. He had never held down a job for more than a month or two, and he had had no employment for years. He took antidepressants when he was very depressed, but rarely continued them for very long, because they did not prevent depression from returning. He could see no route out of his miserable existence.

Dr Ashton suggested to Vince that, although he believed that his problems were intractable, he had asked for help, and that this meant they had to work for change. She acknowledged that it was implausible to suppose that a simple intervention would resolve everything. She suggested that they work together over some time to find solutions to specific problems in order to see whether he could gain control over his life and achieve a more meaningful existence. Over a period of time, this might make life worth living. Vince, sullen though he seemed, said he thought this sounded logical, and he was prepared to give it a try.

Dr Ashton saw Vince monthly for almost a year. It was not a smooth ride. It took time for them to form a comfortable therapeutic relationship. He was often negative about ideas she offered, but sometimes acted on them later. There were episodes of drunkenness, though no self-harm. They examined strategies to contain his binge drinking, and this slowly came under control. Vince came to accept that antidepressants might be more effective if he did not drink, and he started to take them regularly. He enrolled in night classes to get some qualifications, and it turned out that he had a flair for computers.

Vince and Dr Ashton reviewed the situation after twelve months. He was still chronically unhappy, and he was far from certain that he would ever get the life that he wanted. Nonetheless, he had to acknowledge that life was better than it had been. He enjoyed his night classes, and he had started talking to another man who also attended. His drinking binges were less frequent and protracted, and he had avoided severe depression. Over the next year, they met less frequently, and focussed on problems as they arose, looking for new ways of dealing with them. He formed a close friendship with the man at the night class. He found temporary employment covering sickness in an IT department of a department store, and when this ended he was offered a permanent part-time job. This suited him, because the hours were short, and there was limited contact with other employees.

Reviewing treatment at the end of the second year, Vince surprised Dr Ashton by saying that he wanted to be discharged. She had, he said, done what she said she would. His life was better now, and he had brought some specific problems under control. He now had some choices. He could see a way forward, but there was a substantial risk that the improvement would not persist, in which case he would kill himself. After all her help, it would not be fair to do this whilst he was still under follow-up. It was now up to him, and he preferred to go it alone. It was an odd way to acknowledge her help, but she could accept his fundamental logic. At this stage, his life would either move forward under the momentum of the changes that had already happened, or it would not, in which case her intervention had failed. It was unlikely that suicide could be avoided by pressing him to stay in follow-up, so she discharged him.

Some years later, Dr Ashton bumped into Vince at the department store. She said hello and he awkwardly acknowledged her, moving on quickly without further exchange. She noticed that his name badge said 'Assistant Manager, IT'.

development. The latter corresponds to frank personality disorder. It is important to recognise that mental illness can be an extreme circumstance that exposes problems in someone with an otherwise normal personality.

One cannot locate personality solely in behaviour, and the intervening mechanism between a narrowed behavioural repertoire and a difficult childhood is internal experience. This includes difficulties with attachment, poor self-esteem, insecurity, intolerance of adverse emotion, chronic anger, impulsivity and emotional lability. Nonetheless, thinking about personality problems in terms of behavioural repertoire can sometimes help find a way forward in ordinary clinical settings. There are specific treatments for some personality problems, including therapeutic communities, dialectical behaviour therapy and psychodynamic psychotherapies. However, it would be neither practical nor desirable to refer all patients with personality problems or personality disorders for these interventions. There is a good deal that can and should be done in the context of generic mental health treatment.

Helping people to overcome personality problems requires patience and persistence. Within the setting of general adult psychiatry it tends to turn on finding small steps that help people to deal with particular difficulties differently, and hence extending their behavioural repertoire. This in turn has an impact on the way they feel about themselves. Change tends to be slow, and it is rarely dramatic. No one can turn into a completely different person. Over time, however, people can change what they do to a surprising extent.

Whilst it is rarely appropriate to use specific psychotherapeutic techniques for treatment of personality disorder outside of a specialist setting, a degree of sophistication in one's understanding of personality development is helpful. There is a large literature on borderline personality disorder and psychopathic personality that is useful in this regard, but it is important to recognise that a high proportion of personality problems that are encountered in general adult mental health practice are obsessional or avoidant in nature. There is a definite skew in thinking about personality problems, whereby services have a strong focus on people whose behaviour causes problems to other people, either because they are heavy users of mental health facilities or because they are antisocial. Where personality problems cause anxiety, avoidance and indecisiveness they can be overlooked. Whilst there is always a danger of misconstruing difficult behaviour as being due to personality factors rather than underlying mental illness, there is an equal problem in failing to recognise that some problems are unequivocally personality based. It is counter-productive to attempt to treat personality problems as if they might be amenable to a simple solution, particularly if this means a search for the 'right' combination of medications. Bearing in mind that personality problems and mental illness often co-exist, it takes careful judgement to work out the relationship between the two and the most productive way forward. This can only be achieved with the patient working as a partner in the exercise, and with a willingness to reconsider one's ideas in the face of evidence that treatment is not proceeding well. There are no simple solutions or rigid rules that can be applied, and the test of whether one has got it right is the extent to which people are helped to change.

There are some well-recognised pitfalls in treating people with major personality problems. These include:

- *Failing to maintain boundaries.* Maintenance of professional boundaries is always important, but they are particularly challenged when working with people whose personality problems affect their ability to form and maintain appropriate relationships. Becoming overinvolved and trying to rescue people or becoming hostile and punitive are just two of the common ways in which things go wrong.
- *Failing to establish shared treatment objectives.* People with personality problems who are antisocial can use psychiatric treatment as a way of escaping from the consequences of their actions, under the guise of seeking help. A degree of skepticism (but not cynicism) over motivations is justified when people ask for help against the backdrop of criminal proceedings. This means taking particular care in the process of identifying clear treatment aims. Properly done, this will usually expose ulterior motives where they exist.
- *Open-ended treatment.* Treatment that has no recognisable end point can easily become fruitless or part of the person's cycle of maladaptive behaviour. It can be avoided through clear objective setting and periodic joint review of progress.

- *Over- and undertreatment of mental illness.* People with personality disorders who are depressed respond to antidepressants much as other people do. Antipsychotic medication can be surprisingly helpful in people who are chronically emotionally overaroused and who feel out of control. Trying to use medication as the primary focus of treatment, however, is rarely helpful.
- *Using inpatient treatment as a key component of treatment.* Ordinary inpatient units do not offer a constructive therapeutic milieu to help people with personality problems, not least because the issues of control that are intrinsic to that setting can cause conflict or dependency. This is not to say that it is always inappropriate to admit people with personality problems. Admissions do need to be brief and to have a clear purpose.
- *Failing to give up when it is not working out.* Persisting in trying to get someone to change when they cannot or will not is not helpful. One has to be willing to accept that some problems have no solution, and to find a constructive way of putting this to the patient.

Whether they recognise it or not, all clinicians spend a significant proportion of their professional lives working with people who have personality problems, and a willingness to engage with personality difficulties makes the task easier for clinician and patient. It seems to us that the key is to understand the nature of the problem, and to be willing to have a plan that is relatively structured and pragmatic. The individual components to this kind of work vary widely, and we could not begin to set them all out here. We have tended to find personality problems less difficult to manage as we have become more experienced, which is probably due to a gradual expansion in our own repertoire of ways of helping people to do things differently. We have also found access to psychotherapeutic consultation invaluable. Talking through these kinds of problems with a psychotherapist has proven more useful than referral of patients to them for treatment.

Is recovery a realistic aim for everyone?

The development of the concept of recovery as a treatment objective has not depended on the emergence of dramatic new treatments. Instead it involves deploying our existing, imperfect treatments within a therapeutic relationship that is different to the old asylum-based model of paternalism. Despite the fact that clozapine has been the only truly novel treatment to emerge in our working lifetimes, we have a firm impression that the outcome of serious mental disorder has changed. Compared to thirty years ago, patients seem to do better and to be less likely to develop the 'burnt-out' syndromes that were prevalent in the old mental hospitals. They seem to be more likely to have a good quality of life in the community and to have a much better chance of being discharged from follow-up. We cannot say whether this impression is accurate. It may be that the impression arises because long-stay facilities are now located far away from acute services and community teams. It may be wishful thinking, arising from a personal need to believe that our involvement in service development has made a difference. Even bearing these possibilities in mind, the impression remains with us.

We are certain that we are doing less harm than we were, because overmedication and unnecessary incarceration have sharply decreased. However, some people still are burdened by long-term disability and illness, and some illnesses still follow a deteriorating course. Bipolar affective disorder can become a lot more unstable as people approach their seventh and eighth decades.

Bearing this in mind, is recovery a realistic objective for everyone with mental illness? If some people are unlikely to experience symptomatic improvement, could it be that for them recovery is unachievable and that setting an unrealistic objective is cruelly tantalising?

Recovery is only likely to occur if you strive for it. The problem with accepting that it is impossible for some people is that this is a self-fulfilling prophecy. There are often different attitudes to people with different disorders, and this has an impact on expectations of them. Professionals tend to be more respectful of the wishes of people suffering from severe affective disorders than they are of the wishes of people suffering from schizophrenia. However, there is no intrinsic difference between the two types of disorders. They are both potentially disabling, they are both prone to recurrence, and they both can lead to suicide. Both can be associated with 'lack of insight' and non-adherence to treatment plans, but in neither case is this commonly insurmountable. People with schizophrenia have just as much right to make their own choices as anyone else, and it is not surprising to find that treatment seems to proceed better when they are encouraged to have control over their own well being.

Recovery is not really about the elimination of symptoms. It was remarkable to be involved in the British deinstitutionalisation programmes, when people with chronic psychotic illnesses who had lived in back wards of mental hospitals for decades were moved out into group homes in the community. Their chronic symptoms did not greatly alter, but their lives did. In their new homes they had choices and involvement in the ordinary pleasures of life. Many seemed to be transformed, though not miraculously 'cured'. They remained to some extent dependant on mental health staff, but nonetheless, they experienced a type of recovery, and it was moving to witness it. Recovery is always a possibility, because even the most intractable illnesses do change with time and, overall, more people's illnesses improve than worsen as they get older. If you believe that chronically ill people can only ever function as they do right now, they always will. Recovery and staying well is not about unrealistic aims or therapeutic heroism. It is about instilling realistic hope and capitalising on opportunities for change as they occur.

Helping people to stay well is difficult because it means trying to involve them in their treatment even when they resist. It means coping with uncertainties and it demands fine judgements as to when enough is enough. It means discharging people who may or may not do well thereafter, because that is what autonomy is all about. It has to include the right to make mistakes.

As we mentioned in Chapter 12, the use of depot antipsychotic medication to prevent relapse in schizophrenia has been a very marked feature of British psychiatry, and a high proportion of all the depot medication manufactured in the world has been given to British patients. Few British psychiatrists have been aware that this reliance on depot preparations is a national idiosyncrasy, though the habit does appear to be on the wane.

There seems to be little doubt that depot medications work well, though their use can be understood as an oppressive method of controlling people or as a legitimate and sensible choice for some people. In our experience, they can be either, depending on the clinician's relationship with and attitude towards the patient. Treatments are rarely intrinsically good or bad, it depends how you use them. It seems to us that this is the central principle in helping people to stay well.

Main points in this chapter

1. If you do not have recovery as an aim you cannot achieve it.
2. The mark of successful treatment is that patients are discharged equipped with the skills necessary to manage their own disorder.
3. Access to professional help when it is needed is more constructive than indefinite dependent follow-up.
4. Helping people to stay well usually involves helping them to overcome a range of contextual difficulties in a pragmatic and stepwise fashion.
5. Helping people to overcome the effects of personality problems is often an intrinsic part of facilitating an enduring improvement in their mental health.
6. Whilst medication may be important in staying well, it is by no means the most important factor.

Part IV – Coping

Some problems have no solution, and you just have to find ways of coping with them. Prominent amongst these are true dilemmas, where all options are unsatisfactory, and the inexorable process of change that is a backdrop to all careers in the mental health services.

17 Coping with dilemmas

True dilemmas arise relatively frequently in day-to-day work in mental health, and they are an important aspect of clinical practice. Dilemmas are not simply difficult decisions. They arise when the clinician is confronted with a choice between two or more unsatisfactory courses of action. It is in the nature of dilemmas that there is no right answer, and that there is no readily available template that can be used to resolve them.

There is an ethical dimension to many clinical dilemmas, which makes matters considerably more complicated. Different ethical imperatives can be in conflict with each other. For example, the principle of respect for patient autonomy can guide decision making towards consequences that conflict with the professional duty to preserve life. Because there are no wholly satisfactory solutions available to resolve dilemmas, the clinician is left feeling uneasy about the course that he has followed. This creates a temptation to shy away from dilemmas, to either refuse to deal with them at all, or to resolve the tension of uncertainty by denying the complexities of the situation. Following the line of least resistance in this way is bound to lead either to default non-decisions or to ill-considered decisions. Invariably these are eventually regretted.

Clinical dilemmas are protean phenomena. They come in a multitude of forms, and even after decades of practice you continue to encounter novel problems of this sort. Although there are no formulae to resolve them, there are two principles that are useful in dealing with them. The first is that you should acknowledge the full nature of the dilemma and draw out exactly what it is that makes decision making difficult in the circumstances. The second is that in deciding what to do, you should clearly identify the reasons for taking the chosen course of action. These processes demand self-discipline. If applied with a degree of candour and openness, they routinely expose the fact that one of the obstructions to decision making is the clinicians' emotional reactions to the situation.

Recording these two processes has a utility in protecting professionals if things should go wrong, but they have a greater importance in facilitating clear thinking. Separating clinicians' emotions from the real issues for the patient is helpful in identifying pseudo-dilemmas. These are situations where spurious clinical arguments are put forward to avoid taking unpalatable but sensible actions. For example, we earlier discussed the fact that legal compulsion is a regrettable but necessary part of psychiatric treatment and that mental health professionals involved in a patient's care cannot distance themselves from it, because teamwork demands that there should be joint ownership of all legitimate aspects of care.

Mental health professionals sometimes decline to involve themselves in legal detention on the grounds that it will undermine their therapeutic relationship with the patient. However, there is no true dilemma here. Professionals may have difficulty in saying unwelcome things to the patient (e.g. 'You are too unwell to safely remain at home and you need to go into hospital') or they may be fearful of unpleasantness or aggression. However, therapeutic relationships are more severely compromised by professionals dishonestly disowning necessary aspects of care than they are by the acknowledgement of unpalatable truths. Indeed, the recognition and exploration of difficult truths is a process that is part of many therapeutically useful relationships. When professionals decline to face these issues, they are undermining their effectiveness and breaching a boundary concerning honesty. It is an unacceptable self-indulgence for clinicians to avoid those parts of their work that they personally find awkward (this is rather different to conscientious objection to the use of compulsion, which is a position that is usually incompatible with taking a professional role within mainstream mental health services).

We shall briefly explore a handful of common dilemmas, some of which have been mentioned or alluded to earlier in the book.

Personal idiosyncrasies

Idiosyncratic practice is a common and difficult problem in psychiatry. This is not just a question of a small number of dangerously opinionated practitioners. In a field where interpersonal skills are as important as technical knowledge, and where treatment technologies have marked limitations, it is not surprising to find that all practitioners have their idiosyncrasies. Experience and personality shape our practice. Diversity is desirable up to a certain point. It encourages innovation and extends the range of treatment that is available. However, the determinedly maverick practitioner is unequivocally a hazard to patients. The difficulty is in deciding where the limits of respectability lie. *I* am a brave and progressive innovator. *You* are an arrogant exponent of quack psychiatry.

Unfortunately, normative tests may not be the best way of evaluating the limits of appropriate and respectable treatment. Some practitioners feel strongly that mainstream psychiatry has drifted too far away from the psychosocial and too far towards the biological. They would argue that this drift is in conflict with the empirical evidence with regards to what works best. Biological treatments may be based on technology, but their dominance is not based on science. The psychosocially orientated practitioner may be at one end of the spectrum of contemporary practice, but he may have a greater fidelity to the historical mission of psychiatry than the practitioner who sits on the mean of present day practice. This is our own belief. Naturally enough, we think we are right. However, we may be wrong, and our intractable attachment to the psychosocial may place us in a far more extreme position with regard to the mainstream than we are prepared to recognise. Who is best placed to make a judgement on these matters?

Changes in the Zeitgeist can move some practitioners from the mainstream to the margins. In the UK, psychoanalytic psychotherapy has experienced a rapid fall from grace. It was never a dominant modality in NHS practice, but it was widely available twenty-five years ago, and it was taken seriously. There are now only a few pockets of traditional psychoanalysis left in the NHS, and it is fair to say that it is no longer generally regarded as a respectable mainstream treatment. This is problematic for that group of psychiatrists of our generation who have always had a strong attachment to psychoanalysis. This orientation was nurtured by the NHS when it trained them. Policy makers now tend to condemn psychoanalysis as unscientific, ineffective and wasteful of resources, especially in the face of the more compelling claims of CBT. If a psychiatrist sincerely feels that the best solution to a patient's problems is traditional psychoanalysis, should they tell the patient, bearing in mind that only a small minority of British psychiatrists would be likely to agree?

We believe that mental health professionals have an obligation to do their best to remain within the discernable parameters of respectable practice. When personal beliefs or other idiosyncrasies take us outside of those parameters, we should make this clear to our patients. It is one thing to give idiosyncratic advice whilst acknowledging that many or most psychiatrists would give different advice. It is quite another to give maverick advice under a false impression of respectability. If there is any resolution to this dilemma, it rests on the maintenance of boundaries, and in particular the rule that forbids professionals from misrepresenting themselves. The alternative (of making the assumption that one's idiosyncratic opinions are necessarily right) usurps the patient's right to understand the nature of the treatment that is being proposed. It puts the professional's needs before the patient's, which is never acceptable.

Unethical policies

Ethical dilemmas are not abstractions, and systematically unethical practice is not a remote hypothetical possibility. Robert Lifton's book *The Nazi Doctors* (Lifton, 1986) is now quite old, and it relates to events that occurred long before most modern psychiatrists were born. Nonetheless it is essential reading. Psychiatrists were deeply involved in the operation of the Nazi death camps, and the interviews in Lifton's book reveal doctors who were discernibly similar to us.

Nazi Germany was not an isolated example of psychiatrists collaborating with unethical government policies. Soviet psychiatrists at the Serbsky Institute in Moscow collaborated with the regime's efforts to reframe dissent as a form of mental illness. They developed a pseudo-scientific concept of 'sluggish schizophrenia' and misused treatments on dissidents in ways that could reasonably be construed as torture (Bloch & Reddaway, 1977). Today, psychiatrists in the USA struggle with the consequences of the nation's continued extensive use of judicial killing. Serious ethical dilemmas are created when psychiatrists are asked to assess prisoners who have been accused of capital crimes. International medical ethical codes forbid doctors from involvement in the death penalty because of the ethical duty to preserve life and to act in the interests of the patient. These duties apply to all doctors, irrespective of their personal opinion about the use of execution. Even if one construes the psychiatrist's role as a positive one (in that a psychiatric defence can save the prisoner's life), the conclusion that the accused was responsible for his actions and that there is no psychiatric defence for the crime may condemn the person to death.

There is an argument that is sometimes used in an attempt to bypass the ethical difficulties concerning forensic psychiatry in general and the death penalty in particular. It is said that the accused is not the patient of the assessing doctor, and therefore the usual ethical framework does not apply. The difficulty with this position is it can be used to justify *any* ethical breach by claiming that one can legitimately move backwards and forwards between acting as a doctor and not a doctor. The *'I'm not acting as a doctor right now'* argument does not resolve the problem. Doctors making assessments as to the applicability of the death penalty (whether this involves criminal responsibility or fitness for execution) can be regarded as carrying out a function similar in ethical category to the medical assessment of prisoners' fitness for forced labour as they disembarked from trains at the Nazi death camps. The latter doctors may have thought they were saving some detainees from extermination, but a more objective judgement suggests that they were deciding who would die.

The 'now-I'm-a-doctor-now-I'm-not' notion is seductive because it appears to neatly resolve a dilemma, but it is actually ethically bankrupt. It illustrates why it is important to continue to understand relationships between medical professionals and service users as doctor–patient relationships, as this framework implicitly sets the relationship within the ambit of a clear set of ethical imperatives.

Serious ethical problems involving the misuse of psychiatry rarely come along as a dramatic departure from normal practice, with a label marked 'caution–may lead to genocide'. Systematic abuses develop in stages, without any clear indication that the situation has moved from the ethically questionable to the ethically unacceptable. This means that mental health professionals have to guard against collaboration with unethical government or institutional policies at all levels of seriousness, no matter how minor they may initially appear.

In the UK there has been a long war of attrition between the government and an alliance of service users, carers and mental health professionals over unethical proposals for reform of mental health legislation. Although the proposals have been whittled down to a less threatening package than was initially proposed, there will be a need for further struggle in the years to come, because the modified proposals remain ethically unacceptable. British forensic psychiatrists have recently found themselves involved in the care of prisoners detained as terror suspects, at risk of indefinite detention, deportation and torture. Serious dilemmas involving conflict between government policy and ethical codes are not remote or hypothetical. They are upon us and they will not go away.

Whom do ethics belong to?

Medical ethics are not unchanging absolutes. They alter according to shifts in prevalent social values. Medical paternalism caused little comment forty years ago, but it has become largely unacceptable. It is rejected by contemporary codes of practice (General Medical Council, 2006). It is right and proper that we should be attentive to alterations in social mores, though it is not always obvious how or where prevalent values are formed. There are particular ambiguities as to the ownership of professional ethical codes. Whom do they really belong to?

The dominant values influencing medical practice are not necessarily the same as, or even similar to, those held by the population at large. For example, the primacy of informed consent and patient choice, predicated on a particular understanding of free will, is taken to be a truism by more or less everyone with an interest in medical ethics, including us. Research ethics committees place great emphasis on informed consent and choice. They apply austere conditions to research that merely inconveniences subjects and that does not risk irreversible alterations in health. Similarly, patient choice has become the pre-eminent guiding principle in reforming the NHS. A type of health care market has been contrived, such that the closure of some local hospitals appears to be a logical inevitability. However, one of the differences between the British and American populations is that the former do not seem to value choice as highly as the latter. On the contrary, there is much to suggest that large sections of the British public are willing to forgo choice in health care if they are offered local services of a decent standard that are accessible and safe. Similarly, it is by no means clear that the general population prefers ethically immaculate research to optimal medical progress. Even if people do, it is quite certain that a substantial proportion of the population does not like being offered too much choice when frightened and in pain. In an emergency, a lot of people prefer medical paternalism.

The reification of choice and consent in health care may have very little to do with the wishes of most people living in the UK. It may have a great deal more to do with a change in ethos whereby health care has traditionally been a *service* (provided by charity or through taxation) but is rapidly becoming a *commodity*. Commodities must be exchanged through the application of free will and choice, or there can be no market. Far from being a patient-centred development, the modern emphasis on choice may actually serve the needs of health care providers as they seek to profit from selling their wares in a free market.

Some conflicts between medical ethics and popular attitudes are more obvious than this. In a democracy, there is a constitutional assumption that the government represents the will of the people. This aspiration may or may not be realised by particular regimes, but it seems to us that government policy corresponds with public opinion in the UK on the matter of mental health. The general public seems to support more restrictive and custodial care for people with mental illnesses. Similarly, it seems that the majority of the people of the UK support capital punishment, more than forty years after it was abolished. Organised medicine (together with the other health professions) does not accept these popular attitudes. We are no exception in this regard. We agree that health professionals cannot be involved in processes leading to judicial execution, and we oppose oppressive mental health legislation. However, this means that we are unequivocally taking the position that it is legitimate for us to hold ethical values that are different to those of the society that we serve. The implication is that society should come into line with us, not vice versa.

None of the above is intended as an attack upon conventional ethics, on research ethics committees or the principle of patient choice. There is no doubt that in the past health professionals (especially doctors) have been far too unaccountable. However, there is a real tension between the legitimate accountability of our professions and the duty of clinicians to stand their ground when they come under pressure to do things that they believe are wrong.

The key point here is that it is not at all clear who has ownership of ethics. The general public, the professions, politicians, patients and the institutions of the establishment all have a claim, but none has primary ownership. Ethically appropriate behaviour is a peculiar combination of responsiveness to social expectations and due regard to what appears to be irreducible and absolute values. Professionals have a duty to avoid proselytising their own beliefs. We have commented on the dangers of idiosyncratic practice. Notwithstanding these imperatives, the fact is that the ultimate ethical test is that you must remain true to yourself. It is common experience that one most often regrets those actions that are taken in betrayal of the personal duty to do what you think is right.

Difficult families

The concept of the 'difficult family' is awkward. 'Difficult' often means articulate and demanding, which may be tiresome for the professional, but is perfectly reasonable from the family's point of view. Some families are more troublesome than this. It is not so much that they challenge professionals' ideas. They do things that are objectively counter-productive to the task of getting the patient better. For the most part these difficult families are ordinary people who are stressed by extraordinary circumstances. Although misguided, they are trying to help the patient or to control difficult feelings of their own. Working with families like this is part of the bread and butter of everyday clinical intervention.

Truly difficult problems with families are less common. From time to time you come across severely dysfunctional family configurations, where progress is almost impossible because of family factors. This can be due to psychopathology in another family member. For example, in cases of folie à deux a second family member resists treatment for the index patient in the belief that the delusions are true. Similarly, some relatives cannot accept that the patient has a mental illness (because of shame or some other emotional reaction of their own) and they aggressively collude with the evasion of treatment, sometimes to the point of attempted legal action. Still more difficult, some families or family members are just plain bad. Because mental illness can affect anyone, it is inevitable that some relatives prove to be malign or unpleasant people who behave in ways that are reprehensible. For example, we had the experience of treating an extremely vulnerable young woman whose partner preferred that she remained psychotic because she was more compliant with his unusual sexual preferences when unwell.

One's natural response when confronted with these situations is to feel that the patient would be better off without the offending relatives. The clinician has a strong urge to cut them out of the treatment process and perhaps to eliminate them from the patient's life. Of course, under most circumstances this far exceeds the limits of legitimate intervention. Families, no matter how dysfunctional or unpleasant, cannot be replaced. Only patients can make a choice to turn their back on them. Partners are chosen, and patients have just as much right to make bad choices in this matter as in any other.

Here is a true dilemma. Should you work with unpleasant people who have no intention of pulling in the same direction as you? Working on the relationship with a dysfunctional family may help it to become more functional. This is usually the right thing to do, but not always. Sometimes you come to feel that you are colluding with deviant behaviour and that the patient is suffering as a consequence. Sometimes you have to very firmly confront and oppose malevolent or seriously misguided relatives. Unfortunately, we have yet to find a way of reliably deciding which is the best course of action. We have made errors in both directions, including a memorable case where the patient was eventually found drowned in a canal following a drunken fight with her abusive partner, who could not remember how he came to be separated from her on the night in question.

The other true dilemma involving families concerns situations where there is a conflict of interests between the patient and a family member who is more vulnerable than the patient. This generally concerns spouses or patients' parents.

Such situations are not rare. Ambiguities and complexities are the rule, which makes it very difficult to know what to do for the best. All that we can recommend is our earlier advice to identify and record the nature of the dilemma and the reasons for the decision made, so that you can at least be sure that a positive and considered decision has been made, rather than throwing up one's hands in despair and avoiding doing anything at all.

Quick fixes

From time to time clinicians come under pressure to take expedient action that will resolve an immediate problem, but which is counter-productive or wrong in the longer run. A key example is to admit a patient to an inappropriate setting when it is difficult to secure a specialist bed. This is not to argue for pedantic rigidity over the type of patient that can be cared for in general adult psychiatric units. A wide range of people can be appropriately cared for in this setting. There is no reason to exclude anyone unless the staff lack the specific skills needed to care for them adequately or they are likely to be very vulnerable there. It is not uncommon for general adult psychiatrists to be asked to admit psychotic children (i.e. aged fifteen years or less) to adult wards because of the very sparse provision of specialist child psychiatry beds. Complying with the request relieves everyone's anxieties, but one usually comes to regret the decision. Similar problems are caused by requests to admit people with such a severe learning disability that they lack speech. These requests usually include the promise that a specialist bed will soon be available and that the admission will be for a few days at the most.

It can feel very uncomfortable to resist such requests, because one is aware that patients and their families are distressed. Resistance can seem unfeeling and certainly unhelpful. Sometimes acquiescing to such requests is the right thing to do, or simply the only choice available. However, holding out for a proper solution sometimes serves patients' interests better. Children and severely learning disabled adults can be extremely vulnerable to bullying and exploitation on adult wards. Ordinary ward staff find it hard to assess and treat them appropriately. There is an understandable pressure to overuse medication in order to eliminate unfamiliar behaviour patterns. The 'few days' promise is rarely honoured, because the whole system loses all sense of urgency once the patient is 'safely' in a hospital bed. Alternative (if expensive) arrangements are sometimes made surprisingly quickly if one sticks to a reasonable refusal to do the expedient but wrong thing.

Pressure to use compulsion to resolve an irresolvable problem is another example of the quick fix. In the case of Brendan set out in Box 17.1, one can well imagine that his mother might ask for him to be admitted to hospital under compulsion to get him off drugs (which would be neither legal nor effective) or a well-meaning and forceful relative of the pair pressing for Brendan to be admitted in order to reduce the risk (which would allay concerns in the short run, but would ultimately fail because resolving psychotic symptoms would be unlikely to alter risk to any substantial extent). Yet another type of quick fix arises when patients want to use treatment facilities for non-therapeutic or counter-therapeutic ends, such as being admitted to avoid situational difficulties such as legal proceedings, or being given benzodiazepines to extinguish normal emotional reactions. It seems perfectly clear that quick fixes are to be avoided, but one has to acknowledge that the pressure to utilise them can be intense.

One cannot propose a rule that quick fixes are never appropriate, not least because what appears to be a quick fix can occasionally have an unexpected and enduring effect for the better. However, the rule around quick fixes (in keeping with dilemmas in general) is to be clear as to the likely consequences and as to whether the overall situation is likely to improve for the patient once the immediate crisis has passed.

Unacceptable choices

Patients need dignity, respect and autonomy. They need to be able to make choices, even if they are bad ones. Clinicians should understand and respect patients' cultures and values. These are important principles which we would like to think we adhere to. It is true that choices in state-funded services can be extremely limited, but even then, these principles drive aspirations for the future. However, there is a problem when patients want to make choices that we find unacceptable or personally offensive.

Some patients do not want to be treated by clinicians from a different ethnic group. This is sometimes, but not always, a consequence of racist bigotry that is utterly unacceptable to people working in the essentially liberal professions of the mental health services. People from some religious groups are antagonistic to homosexuality and may not wish to be treated by openly gay professionals. Some patients have a strong preference over the gender of the staff they work with, which may reflect emotional sensitivities, religious belief or sexism.

If people have strong preferences, it seems wrong to dismiss them. However, pandering to bigotry also seems wrong. It is surely horribly paternalistic and patronising to have a different response to such preferences depending on whether we consider the motivation behind them to be legitimate. Ignoring such preferences might appear to

---

Box 17.1 Whose welfare comes first?

At the age of fifty-three, Brendan had been a committed drug user for some thirty-five years. He was physically dependent on opiates, but he actually preferred stimulant drugs. Heavy smoking, combined with years of inhaling cannabis and crack cocaine, had caused emphysema. A road accident in his thirties had left him with brain injury and a degree of frontal lobe impairment.

Brendan had had an admission to mental hospital with schizophreniform symptoms when he was nineteen, long before his drug use had become seriously out of control. Thereafter he had been prone to psychotic symptoms, which tended to accompany stress and heavy stimulant misuse. His psychosis was adequately controlled by a depot antipsychotic. There was agreement within the CMHT that schizophrenia was probably the least of his problems.

Brendan lived with his widowed mother. Although she had coped with his drug use for many years, she could not accept it. Undeterred by three decades of failure, she continued to try to persuade Brendan to stop taking drugs by an act of will. Since his brain injury, she controlled his money. She hid his drugs, prescribed and recreational, and administered them according to an erratic regime of her own invention. For the most part Brendan could live with his mother's scheme. From time to time there were terrible rows, either because her regime pushed Brendan into opiate withdrawal or because she found his reserve stash of street drugs. Sometimes during these rows her frustration would drive her to hit him with a rolling pin, showing a punitive vigour that was surprising in a woman of advanced years.

Although Brendan and his mother cared for each other, the CMHT feared that his mother was at risk of being seriously injured or even killed. Mostly the arguments involved a lot of shouting. However, when she assaulted him, his efforts to defend himself could be clumsy. On several occasions he had pushed her away too hard and she had fallen. On one occasion she had broken her collarbone. When Brendan was experiencing symptoms of psychosis and opiate withdrawal he could be very irritable. It seemed obvious that it was only a matter of time before all the circumstances would converge into a serious injury. Brendan and his mother were dismissive of these concerns, and neither one was prepared to take any action to reduce the tensions between them.

The CHMT found it extremely difficult to decide what to do. On the one hand, Brendan's mother was seventy-seven years old and she was frail. On the other hand, Brendan's mental illness made only a small contribution to the overall risk. His mother played a significant role in creating the risk, and she rejected advice aimed at securing her safety. If the CMHT intervened, for example, to separate them, neither would be pleased. Separating them could be seen as putting the mother's best interests first. She was, however, mentally well, whilst he had two mental health problems (excluding addiction). If she came to harm, so would Brendan, if only through being sent to prison. It was hard to decide which of them was the most vulnerable.

be the right course of action, but it creates other problems. Is it fair to expect a black professional to work with a patient who expresses white supremacist attitudes or who is otherwise racially offensive?

It is not the job of the clinician to proselytise any personal opinion, but clinicians do have some rights. Just as people cannot be expected to tolerate being threatened or assaulted in the course of their work, they cannot be expected to tolerate persistent behaviour that they find offensive. It would be wrong to try to change a white supremacist's mind. On the other hand, it is quite reasonable to explain that you find their views offensive and that if they continue to express those views in the setting of mental health treatment, the effectiveness of the treatment is bound to be adversely affected. Whether or not it is right to conform to bigoted preferences, it is generally not possible. Mental health professionals are not available in such abundance and diversity to provide everyone with a clinician with the 'right' profile.

Fortunately, bigotry tends to retreat in the face of human relationships. Getting to know someone from the group you are prejudiced against can have a powerful impact in changing ideas. When this does not happen, the professional has to retain the right to decline to work with a patient who is prejudiced against them. This may create problems in delivering an optimal service, but some problems have no solution.

This is not the only area where clinicians' choices are as legitimate as patients' choices. Patients sometimes decide they want to change their CMHT key worker. Although it is right to be attentive to patients' preferences, the search for a new key worker can be counter-therapeutic. It can represent an attempt to find someone with less secure boundaries. It can be part of a pattern of habitual querulant complaint. The patient may be in search of someone who is supportive of a generous attitude to the prescribing of abusable drugs such as hypnotics. The decision as to whether to comply with these requests involves balancing patients' reasonable expectation of choice with the need for clinicians to retain responsibility for the therapeutic effectiveness of the intervention. This is best achieved through team discussion. An individual decision is more likely to be capricious or otherwise inappropriate.

Treating colleagues

Doctors are notorious for neglecting their health. Mental health professionals, sad to say, can be extraordinarily reluctant to acknowledge that they have a mental health problem themselves. They worry about confidentiality and they tend to have very strong preferences over who they will allow to treat them. They struggle with the transition from clinician to patient, and this can make them very difficult to assess. It is extremely difficult to persuade psychiatrists to describe their mental health problems without an intrusive degree of interpretation and self-diagnosis. On top of all this, there are realistic obstructions to securing psychiatric help for health professionals, because they often have prior relationships with clinicians that preclude an appropriate therapeutic relationship.

Psychiatrists, and to a lesser extent other health professionals, have a relatively high suicide rate. There are excellent reasons to make it as easy as possible for colleagues to get psychiatric treatment when they need it, and this can mean going outside of the normal systems. Set against this is a powerful and invariable law of psychiatry: Special Cases Are Bad Cases. This is such an important law that we suggest readers memorise it. The usual systems work reasonably well most of the time. The more you move outside of them, and the more you compromise over boundaries, the more likely it is that things will go wrong. The reasons for special arrangements are usually cogent but they are relatively unimportant in the face of their strong tendency to drive a therapeutic intervention into dysfunctionality and failure.

Clearly the imperatives of making it as easy as possible for people to get help whilst trying to stick to the normal ways of doing things are in conflict with each other. We have extensive experience with these situations. We strongly recommend that if a colleague must be taken on out of area, or some other compromise made in order to allow him to get help, this should be the only compromise with normal working. The first negotiation of the therapeutic relationship should be over your insistence that everything else should be done in the normal way. This includes keeping full records within a standard set of case notes.

Is this the best we can do?

There is a continuous tension in clinical practice between doing too little and doing too much for patients suffering from chronic psychosis. There is a group of patients who are settled, but with a poor quality of life. These patients are uncomplaining and make few demands on the service, and they often express complete satisfaction with what appears to be a rather empty and unsatisfying lifestyle. It is extremely difficult to know whether to intervene or not and, if so, how to time this. There is a real risk of destabilising the situation, and well-meaning efforts to improve someone's quality of life can result in relapse, or a series of relapses. Apparently barren lives can be richer than they appear. Apparently irrational medication regimes and emotional understimulation can prove to be critical factors in maintaining the person's well being. Once the situation unravels, it can be difficult to regain stability. On the other hand, intervention can have positive results, and patients' quality of life can dramatically improve. Meddlesome intervention and neglectful inaction are both real risks, and there is little to guide the clinician away from either pitfall. Although experience and careful evaluation are important, they do not prevent you from making mistakes in either direction.

There is another group of people for whom vigorous intervention over years seems to make little or no difference. In Chapter 3 we said that psychiatrists should not attempt to treat conditions where they have little or nothing to offer. This was stated with reference to establishing objectives at the outset of treatment. However, in the fullness of time it can become apparent that treatment has achieved little or nothing. Is it reasonable then to give up? Is it reasonable for someone who is paranoid but not greatly at risk to have no support from mental health professionals? Is it reasonable to abandon someone with a mental illness when their misuse of alcohol prevents all therapeutic progress? If we give up on people when they fail to get better, who should they turn to? On the other hand, what is the point of wasting limited resources on someone who is gaining no discernible benefit? Just to complicate matters, when you do give up, some people deteriorate quite sharply. You are then driven to the conclusion that you were achieving more than you supposed. Should you then return to the status quo ante?

In attempting to resolve these dilemmas, should clinicians rely primarily on patients' opinions? A senior social care manager recently told us that 'service users always know what's best for them', and insisted that this principle had no exceptions. Whilst we sympathised with the underlying sentiment (that patients have been marginalised and ignored in the past, and that their opinions and wishes should be central to the work of mental health professionals), we had to disagree. People seek help from mental health services precisely because they do not know what to do for the best. They are usually frightened and unable to see a way forward. Herein lies the key dilemma in psychiatry; that one has to find a way of getting alongside patients without dominating them, a way of respecting their views without colluding with delusional beliefs or misguided ideas about what is likely to be helpful, and a way of controlling them through legal detention and institutional care without breaking their spirit and inflicting secondary handicaps.

Conclusion

We have explored a very limited range of dilemmas in clinical practice. We have offered no solutions, because if such solutions were available, they would not be dilemmas. Dilemmas just keep coming, and the most important tools in dealing with them are clarity of thought, independent mindedness and an awareness of the ethical implications of day-to-day practice. Although it is perfectly possible to offer patients high-quality treatment under most circumstances, no one ever suggested that mental health practice was easy. The fact that the work is intellectually and personally demanding is one of its great attractions.

Main points in this chapter

1. Dilemmas arise when all courses of action have major drawbacks. This is not uncommon in mental health practice.
2. It is helpful to identify and record the full nature of such dilemmas and the reasons for the chosen course of action.
3. Personal integrity demands that clinicians ensure that they do not drift over the boundary between respectable and maverick practice.
4. It is unlikely that we will ever work in an environment where the unethical misuse of psychiatry is no longer a risk.
5. There are very difficult dilemmas over expedient decisions, over working with impossibly difficult family members and over the tension between therapeutic heroics and complacent neglect.
6. Special Cases Are Bad Cases.
7. Ultimately, some problems have no solution.

18   Coping with change

No one can expect to avoid the transition from young, promising and open-minded specialist to reactionary, outdated and oppositional senior professional. These changes happen slowly and it seems inevitable that you will be the last to notice what has happened. It may be a little paranoid for us to worry that in private our trainees say 'Apparently he was regarded as a skilled and progressive clinician when he was young!' whilst others shake their heads in amazement. However, we cannot be the only aging psychiatrists with concerns that we might be past our best. The neurotic worries of late middle age lack an intuitive salience early in one's career. However, you are set on the route to dysfunctionality and unhappiness long before the relevance of learning to cope with change becomes obvious. It may be wise to think about some of the issues early on.

One of the marked features of being young is that the years appear to pass slowly. The world seems stable, and change is gradual. Although middle age is a much longer phase of life, its years pass with alarming speed, which creates an unmistakable sense that one is hurtling towards old age, infirmity and death. As you get older, the world seems to change at an accelerating pace, and few certainties remain. There are a number of explanatory theories about this universal phenomenon of the perception of accelerating time. These include the idea that we experience each unit of time as a proportion of total time lived (at 5 years of age, one year is 20% and hence a long time, whereas at 50 one year is 2% and therefore a short time) and the idea that memorable milestone events are frequent in youth and infrequent in later life, creating increasing problems in measuring the passage of the years.

The perception of accelerating change is independent of the objective rate of change around us. In all probability the last decade or so really has been a period of unusually rapid change in mental health services, but the belief that we will eventually reach a distant shore of stability is a forlorn hope. One can say with some certainty that change is the one fixed feature of a working life in the field of mental health. The subjective perception of accelerating change dictates that, for most of us, the intrinsically shifting nature of our work is increasingly difficult to cope with.

This is not to say that the problems created by change are illusory. On the contrary, they are very real and they affect everyone involved in mental health care, professionals and services users alike. Clinicians who do not have strategies for coping with change end up burnt-out, anachronistic and incompetent. We have to accept the inevitability of change and we have to have ways of thinking about it that lead to adaptive strategies. We also need a bottom line that is informed by values that are of fundamental importance, because some changes affront these values, in which case we are ethically obliged to resist.

Routes to burn-out

Psychiatrists tend to have conservative attitudes. They do not like alterations in clinical practice and they tend to regard changes to organisational structures as irrelevant and tiresome. It is true that there is a sub-group of psychiatrists who have a bright-eyed faith in reinventing their profession. They relish and embrace change, provided it corresponds to their own ideas and aspirations. However, neither 'conservatives' nor 'progressives' necessarily cope with change well. Coping with change means abandoning cherished working practices and having the humility to accept that someone else may have come up with a better way of doing things. This is difficult for senior professionals to swallow. Failing to cope with change is a major factor leading to 'burn-out', which is a constellation of cynicism, disengagement and emotional exhaustion. Burn-out is common. It is worth trying to avoid it, because it does nothing to improve your effectiveness and it makes you unhappy.

There are two positions that clinicians commonly adopt in the face of change that are particularly likely to prove maladaptive. The first is the position of solitary resistance. This is the classic posture of NHS consultants, and it causes much exasperation. It tends not to work very well, because the organisation has had to find ways of overcoming it. Essentially, when the psychiatrist is confronted with a proposed change, he insists that there is nothing wrong with existing practices, or, in a more sophisticated version, acknowledges that existing practices are not perfect but insists that they are the optimal compromise between a range of conflicting imperatives. Psychiatrists tend to rely on a combination of professional status and scientific evidence to support their case. The understanding of scientific methodology was once the exclusive preserve of doctors, but now that a much wider group of health professionals are comfortable with data analysis, you cannot depend on the other side to lack a grasp of scientific methodology and/or an inclination to check the literature.

The position of solitary resistance can be appropriate, provided the case is sound, which usually means that the evidence has to say what you claim it says. The problem with this position arises when it is repetitive and habitual, and used to resist all perceived threats to the status quo. Some externally initiated changes prove, in the fullness of time, to be improvements. Clinicians have to change in order to retain up-to-date skills. No one can rely for the whole of a career upon a set of professional skills that were acquired as a trainee. Anyone that did so would inevitably have skills that were thirty years out of date at the point of retirement. Resistance is not always wrong, but there is only ever any point in resisting particular changes for specific reasons. The habitual deployment of the solitary resistor posture places the clinician in a state of continuous warfare with the employing organisation. Conflict with managers and colleagues is a much more potent source of stress and unhappiness than clinical work. Because the pressure for change is remorseless, the resistance strategy is bound to fail most of the time. Continuous conflict and recurrent failure are an unhappy combination. It is better to resist that which must be resisted and to accept that which can be tolerated.

The second maladaptive response is to become a heroic leader of change. This position involves accepting the need for, or the inevitability of, change and taking a personal responsibility for making it work. Heroic leaders have broad shoulders and are seen to cope in the face of problems and pressure. They maintain morale through their positive can-do attitude. They lead by example. When change causes an increase in workload, they shoulder the burden. Heroic leaders make life easier for everyone else, because they make sure that things get done and the centre of effort is clearly located within them.

Whilst leading by example can be important in initiating change and establishing credibility for new ways of doing things, it has the weakness of undermining teamwork and broad ownership of change. For the leaders themselves, the position is brittle and hard to sustain. It can become a trap with no easy means of escape because relinquishing the leadership role can feel like letting everyone down. Everyone has limitations. Heroic leaders come under great pressure, but it is difficult for them to acknowledge that they feel overburdened. They are vulnerable to suddenly becoming unable to function. This tends to be a 'last straw' phenomenon, often in response to a relatively small perturbation such as a complaint or an interpersonal difficulty. Once the illusion of invulnerability is broken, it cannot be put back together, and the heroic leader cannot return to that function. Having become the pivotal person that everyone else relies upon, the whole team is then compromised.

Embracing change is often the most adaptive strategy, not least because it creates opportunities to shape the future. However, this is best done as a team effort. Trying to lead change by force of personality is a route to early retirement.

Physician heal thyself

Even when you want to change the way that you do things, alterations in working practices can be surprisingly difficult to initiate and sustain. There are all kinds of powerful psychological and situational forces that drag you back to the familiar and the comfortable. It is difficult to change by an act of will. It is far easier to change by altering structures, settings and timetables. If you want to change what you do, you need to change the systems that you work within.

The work of developing mental health services takes time, and there is in any case a tendency for clinicians to stay in senior posts for very long periods. Clinical work becomes substantially easier as you get to know the patients really well and as you develop an intimate knowledge of your patch. However, there are drawbacks to staying in a job for a long time. You start to have a strong emotional investment in the fortunes of the service, and there is a blurring of the distinction between what is good for the service and what is good for you personally. Over time it becomes more difficult to bear the retreats and compromises that are bound to arise in the face of shifting demands and priorities. Changing your job can have a remarkably positive effect on your attitude to work, even if the difficulties within the new job are as bad as, or worse than, the problems of the old job. We can testify to the positive effects of this from personal experience, and we do not believe that our experience is unusual. There are many salient reasons to stick with one job for a career, not least the powerful bond of the familiar. However, we

---

Box 18.1 Punctuality restored

Dr Pyke was habitually late for everything. He arrived at clinics late, he constantly fielded telephone calls and he worked into the evening, long after everyone else had gone home. His lateness affected everyone else. Patients were kept waiting, so they did not bother to be punctual for appointments, which exacerbated the culture of running late. Other team members were routinely kept waiting. No one was happy.

After a showdown with the rest of the team, Dr Pyke tried to be more punctual. He developed an increased sense of urgency, which made him feel stressed. In his effort to get to appointments on time, he acquired some speeding tickets and a number of endorsements on his driving licence. He was, however, just as late as ever.

The team secretary eventually took the initiative to restore punctuality. 'The trouble with you,' she told him, 'is that you don't ever say no. You're overcommitted, and you try to cope by putting too much in your diary. There are no breaks and there is no time for travelling. You're not just late, you are tired and inefficient as well.'

She took his diary away from him. Only the secretary was now allowed to book things into it. He was forbidden from taking on new commitments without consultation regarding the implications for the rest of the team.

This worked. Dr Pyke relaxed, achieved more during the working day and started arriving home earlier. The rest of the team saved time, and the patients became more punctual because they found it was reciprocated. Eight months later, his wife left him.

---

have found that an occasional move is an excellent protection against burn-out and the long count down to retirement ('Seven years, four months, sixteen days and two hours to go').

New treatments

In Chapter 13 we described personal prescribing algorithms, a habitual pathway of one's personal prescribing repertoire through which alterations in medication proceed in the event of an inadequate response to treatment. New pharmacological, psychological and social treatments continue to be introduced, which create a problem for clinicians in deciding whether and how a new treatment should be incorporated. Pharmaceutical sales representatives recognise that psychiatrists range from volatile prescribers, who can be easily persuaded to use new medications, to stable prescribers, who are very reluctant to change their prescribing habits. Neither position is intrinsically preferable. What is needed is a rational approach to new treatments.

There is a real dilemma as to the most appropriate attitude to the pharmaceutical industry. It is unrealistic to expect to stand entirely aloof from the industry in the hope that corruption can thus be avoided. Modern medications would not exist without the industry, and it has a very long reach. Nearly all aspects of medicine are now affected by pharmaceutical company sponsorship and influence. It can be important to know

---

Box 18.2 One possible approach to new drugs

1. *Only change prescribing if you need to.* Prescribing algorithms should only be changed with caution and on the basis of good evidence that the new treatment is better than the one that it is replacing. The existence of a new treatment is not in itself sufficient justification to use it.
2. *Wait and see.* The usefulness and problems associated with new drugs normally become evident in the first eighteen months on the market. It is as well to wait at least this long before starting to prescribe the medication yourself.
3. *Test the science.* If you are going to take any notice of scientific claims for a drug, you should not rely on the company's interpretation of data. You should insist on being shown published papers, and should be prepared to intellectually test the claims to destruction. This is a good way of retaining critical appraisal skills, but also routinely exposes false inferences; for example, the assumption that reduced side effects will necessarily lead to better treatment adherence.
4. *Be systematic.* Never agree to 'give it a try' and then discuss the result with a representative. This creates an irrational and rhetorical approach to the introduction of new treatments. If you decide to use a new medication, use it systematically for long enough to gain a reliable impression of its effects and drawbacks.

---

about the claims that companies are making for their products, as patients are frequently aware of these claims. On the other hand, contact with representatives exposes you to pharmaceutical promotion, which is not a good guide to rational prescribing. Promotional material can be very selective in its use and interpretation of research data. It is naive to suppose that one is impervious to techniques of persuasion that are successful in influencing the prescribing behaviour of the profession as a whole.

One of us does not see pharmaceutical representatives at all. The other has a fixed diary slot for them, and will meet representatives from any company that requests an interview. We believe that both policies can be justified. However, both of us follow the policy set out in Box 18.2 in deciding whether to change our prescribing algorithm.

We do not suggest that this approach is the only (or even necessarily the most) appropriate policy. It does rely on the existence of other, less cautious clinicians who try new medications with their patients before we are prepared to do so. Following this policy has meant that our patients have not been exposed to some medications that have proven to be problematic, but it also has meant there was a significant delay before they were exposed to some other drugs. One of us was slow to start using clozapine, which arguably delayed a significant health improvement for some patients. Nonetheless, we believe that it is important to have a thought-through policy of some description, in order to avoid drugs appearing and disappearing from one's prescribing repertoire in an arbitrary way.

The unrelenting activity of the pharmaceutical industry creates a risk that you succumb to a faddishly unstable pattern of prescribing. In contrast, in the case of non-pharmacological treatments the danger is that one never adopts them, because no commercial interest is pressing you to do so. New non-pharmacological treatments are difficult to implement, because once the evidence is secure for their effectiveness, clinicians need training and time to use the intervention. Teams have to adjust to making new approaches part of the life of the team. This requires a team culture that is open and scientifically aware. Trying to use new techniques in isolation from the rest of the team rarely works.

Emergent disorders

DSM IV and ICD-10 have contributed to the development of a consistent international psychiatric language, but they have done nothing to eliminate shifts in diagnostic habits and the development of new clinical concepts. On the contrary, it is likely that they have contributed to changes in nosology. They certainly have had to reflect the most noticeable trend in psychiatry over the past twenty-five years whereby problems that were previously regarded as psychological and/or social in origin are now understood by many psychiatrists to be biological problems.

Clinicians of all generations have had to deal with revisions to the understanding of human behaviour, and this is an understandable consequence of continuing scientific endeavour. What is altogether more difficult is the emergence of new disorders of uncertain validity, such as Attention Deficit Hyperactivity Disorder in adults and Chronic Fatigue Syndrome. By definition, the scientific evidence over these emergent disorders is ambiguous, which creates problems for clinicians. One can neither fully embrace nor completely reject these new disorders as valid clinical entities. Ideas over treatment tend to be sharply divided, but one has to somehow find a way of helping the patient anyway. This can be difficult if the patient has a prior attachment to a particular understanding of the problem. A patient who arrives at the psychiatrist's office with a belief that he has Attention Deficit Hyperactivity Disorder and that he will benefit from stimulant medication may be correct. Unfortunately, there is a significant issue from the outset concerning the clinician's and the patient's beliefs over the nature of the disorder. The rhetorical nature of the interaction creates major problems in deciding the most appropriate way forward. For example, the patient may state that he feels a lot better when he takes amphetamine, and believe that this is evidence in support of the diagnosis. For the clinician the same statement is likely to suggest that the patient is vulnerable to stimulant abuse and that a prescription is not a good idea. There is a solid logic behind both ways of thinking, and they are very difficult to reconcile.

We have no neat solution for the problem of emergent disorders. Some clinicians adopt a firm position of either embracing a new concept or rejecting it. We believe this to be a mistake, as either one or the other is likely to prove wrong in the fullness of time. In any case, psychiatry is built upon foundations of science, and if scientific evidence is equivocal, one can only take a position of agnostic skepticism. This does not help very much in resolving questions such as whether stimulants should be prescribed for inattentive adults. All that one can fall back on is the triangle of forces, the balance of scientific evidence, clinical experience and the clinical situation, which includes consideration of the consequences of doing nothing at all.

What about the patient?

Patients are often in contact with mental health services over long periods of time, either continuously or intermittently. Personnel change on a regular basis. New clinicians are prone to change diagnoses and treatment strategies, which from the patients' point of view can mean a radical reformulation of their problems. This can be seriously confusing. A change of diagnosis from personality disorder to psychosis, or vice versa, is likely to bring with it a major change of attitude over a number of important issues, including people's responsibility for their own actions. Such a change can cause serious problems if it is not properly explained and worked through. Much the same is true when clinical procedures alter. Patients in UK services have seen key workers become care co-ordinators. New types of meetings have been introduced such as Care Programme Approach reviews and section 117 meetings. Alongside these new procedures, there have been successive changes in paperwork, and voluminous documents are given to patients and their families to explain their care. The changes are bewildering and from the service user's point of view it is difficult to understand why they have occurred. Why, for example, are patients asked to sign care plans? Does this commit them to anything? Does it mean that they agree with the care plan? If so, is it meaningful to ask them to sign unless there is clear evidence that they have some choices? What about patients treated under legal compulsion? These matters need to be properly explored with patients and families. Without explanation these changing procedures mystify a process that should be clear, and serve a professional need rather than solving problems for patients.

People who have been treated within the mental health services for decades develop a range of expectations and attitudes which are difficult to change. We may have decided that paternalism has created dependency and secondary handicap, but this is not the fault of people who have been affected by it. We cannot expect them to shrug off the consequences of years of treatment just because our ideas have changed. Some patients can only be treated within an older model of care, because it is too much to expect them to shift at will. Most people can be helped to adjust and move forward, to start to think about the meaning of recovery for them, but this is often a complex and lengthy process. The elimination of old problems can lead to the emergence of new ones. People who have been overmedicated whilst residing in an institution can start to make their own choices when the model of care alters. However, this can cause alarm around them when other people do not like the choices they make, such as becoming sexually active in later life.

The human, physical and policy environment of clinical practice is constantly changing, and somehow we have to try to pursue consistent and coherent plans that work for people and make sense to them. The focus of change management tends to be on the professionals, but we have to recognise how change affects our patients too.

Professional use of euphemisms and neologisms

The emergence of euphemisms and neologisms, along with other alterations in terminology, is a marked feature of change in mental health services. We do not like euphemisms much, because we believe that they obscure meaning. We made this point in Chapter 12, when we defended our continuing use of the word 'compliance'. On the other hand, we do strongly believe that some usages are to be avoided because they suggest attitudes and values that are incompatible with good practice. We strongly believe that describing a person as 'a schizophrenic' or 'a manic-depressive' is entirely inappropriate, because it suggests that the most important thing about them is a mental illness. Although describing a patient as someone suffering from schizophrenia is a little more awkward, it better conveys the true situation. Patients are suffering from an illness. They have not been subsumed by the illness. It is not their defining feature.

Taking care over the use of words is not merely a pedantic concern of the anankastic. There are many situations where conveying a precise meaning is important. Reports for courts and for Mental Health Review Tribunals are good examples. Clinicians have to find words that express what is really meant. Furthermore, the terms that are used have to be meaningful to the intended readership. It is no good using exact terminology if it cannot be understood.

When new expressions are introduced, the test of their validity is whether meaning is improved. There has been a recent example of the introduction of a neologism that has caused real and tangible problems, and has caused us great irritation. Innumerable NHS policy documents and discussion papers refer to '*rising acuity*' amongst patients admitted to psychiatric units. Conventional medical definitions would suggest that this means a general improvement in eyesight. It actually refers to a perception that there is a continuing increase in disturbed behaviour on psychiatric wards. ('Acuity' is presumably used here to avoid the awkward 'acuteness', though 'acute' does not mean 'severe', it means 'of sudden onset'. The expression is truly an etymological dog's dinner.) Rising acuity is an item of faith that is used to justify the move back towards locked doors and more custodial forms of care.

We have yet to see any compelling evidence that there has been an increase in disturbed behaviour on inpatient units in our working lifetime. Wards are smaller than they were, and less disturbed patients are now generally treated at home, so that disturbed patients make up a high proportion of a smaller number of inpatients. Professionals are certainly less tolerant of being exposed to threatening or violent behaviour in the course of their work than was once the case. The techniques used by staff to deal with disturbed patients are now more professional and less aggressive than they were, but there is more paperwork generated by aggressive incidents. It is our impression that, if one takes these factors into account, the degree of disturbance on wards is the same or less than it was twenty-five years ago. The term 'rising acuity', however, sets the question of evidence aside, and implies a recognised and established phenomenon. It seems that it is the natural order of things that acuity, like entropy, can only ever increase.

The term 'rising acuity' is not only a linguistic affront, it is also a barrier to clear thinking about the management of disturbed behaviour. Is there is a rising tide of violence on inpatient units that is beyond the control of mental health services, or are there changes that are primarily a consequence of alterations in the organisation of services? The solutions are different in each case, and by clearly implying the former, the neologism does nothing to move us towards solutions.

The tendency for mental health professionals to generate euphemisms and neologisms is not going to go away just because we disapprove of it. We do suggest, however, that in this one circumscribed area, a stance of habitual resistance is well justified and may be fruitful.

Conclusion

The main strategy for coping with change is to recognise that it is inevitable and that sometimes it is going to be difficult (though rarely catastrophically so). Specific strategies for dealing with particular types of change rest on one's personality characteristics and the context (especially the team context) that you are working within. You have to find your own strategies for yourself, but you can only do so if you recognise that they are bound to be needed. On balance, change is both necessary and exciting. Despite our own bad tempered reactions to a range of changes over the years, we continue to believe that modern mental health services are of a far higher quality than the services we first encountered three decades ago.

Main points in this chapter

1. Change is inevitable and there is nowhere to hide. It appears to accelerate as you get older, which is amongst the factors that makes it increasingly difficult to cope with.
2. Change is best managed as a team effort. Habitual solitary resistance is destructive, but so is the posture of the hero-innovator.
3. Changes in practice work best if they are supported by alterations to structures, timetables, processes and meetings.
4. New treatments should be approached in a systematic and logical way.
5. Emergent disorders create real dilemmas that can only be resolved in the light of the balance of evidence rather than personal belief.
6. Change is difficult for professionals, but still more so for patients and their families.
7. Euphemisms and neologisms are a bad habit that can be overcome.

Afterword: Optimism of the will and pessimism of the intellect

We opened this book with some very firm and unambiguous statements about the state of modern psychiatry. In Chapter 1 we said: 'There is more cause for therapeutic optimism now than at any other time in the history of psychiatry', 'looking back over our lengthy careers in psychiatry what is really striking is a dramatic improvement in the quality of mental health services.' Attentive readers will have noticed that in subsequent chapters, we have condemned or moaned about a wide range of prominent features of modern mental health services, from government policy to the overuse of counselling. If there is any merit in the arguments that we have made, how can we sustain an upbeat expectation of the future of psychiatry as a therapeutic endeavour?

There have been many ignoble episodes in the history of psychiatry. From time to time it has allowed itself to be misused. Its practitioners have sometimes embraced practices that are objectively harmful to people with mental illness. However, we believe that it is possible to identify a legitimate historical mission that psychiatry has followed from its inception in the nineteenth century until today.

Psychiatry came into existence as a consequence of the formation of the asylums. This was a project that aimed to provide humane and rational care for people suffering from mental illness, rescuing them from the abuses of the private madhouses. It is true that the asylums themselves became places of neglect, and sometimes abuse, but psychiatry then played a leading role in taking care out of mental hospitals, into clinics, and on into peoples' own homes. Psychiatry has progressively altered its attitude towards people with mental illness, increasingly recognising that marginalisation and stigmatisation are inappropriate and damaging, and that our patients benefit the most when they are truly partners in our therapeutic efforts. Psychiatry has developed psychotherapies, social interventions and patterns of service delivery that together have brought us to the point where we could, if we had the will, abolish institutional mental health services completely.

We do not suggest that psychiatry can claim exclusive or primary responsibility for the development of progressive and effective mental health services. Many other professions and forces have played key roles, especially, latterly, the service user movement. Nor can we deny that elements within organised psychiatry have resisted each development as it has emerged. We do, however, suggest that the profession has taken an important and distinctive role in moving things forward at each stage. This is the legitimate historical mission of psychiatry, and we believe it is as relevant now as it was two hundred years ago. In invoking this idea we are vulnerable to the accusation that we are trying to redefine psychiatry by emphasising the good bits and disowning the bad bits, but we disagree. We believe that this mission is recognisable to a large proportion of psychiatrists, and that it does embrace the profession's key aspirations.

Psychiatry is fundamentally a project of the Enlightenment. It is based on liberal values, humanitarianism, rationality, independent mindedness and a secular understanding of the world. Post-modernist thinkers have condemned the ideas of the Enlightenment as a European ethnocentric conspiracy, a kind of intellectual imperialism. However, post-modernism has nothing to put in their place. The relativist belief that no set of ideas has any intrinsic worth or claim to special validity seems to us to have created a cult of the irrational. This can be used to justify anything, and it is dangerous.

This is not to say that psychiatry should be mechanistic. Indeed, reductionist/mechanistic thinking has been one of the recurrent errors of psychiatry, which has made it vulnerable to successive waves of eugenic thinking. Richard Dawkins, professor of the public understanding of science at Oxford University, has become the high priest of mechanistic science, but his ideas (e.g. Dawkins, 1987) make many of us who have a strong commitment to science feel uneasy. Zealous faith in grand overarching concepts and a rejection of uncertainty are not good science.

Mental health services face real threats, and some of the ideas that are currently fashionable with health service managers and policy makers seem to us to be seriously misconceived. It has always been thus. In recognising that mental health services have improved, we are not suggesting that everything is tickety-boo. Another component of the legitimate historical mission of psychiatry is to manage these threats, not by heroically brushing them aside (which is not possible), but by retaining a fundamental sense of direction and avoiding retreats to the practices of the past.

A highly placed clinical psychologist recently suggested to us that psychiatry should be abolished. He was of the view that people with mental illness would be better served by clinical psychologists, who could call upon the expertise of general practitioners to deal with medical issues as they arose. Although we, as individuals, were doing a good job, he said, the existence of psychiatry was damaging to people with mental illness, and the entire rotten edifice had to be destroyed. He defended this point of view by reference to Foucault, Szasz and Laing.

In our opinion, Foucault and Szasz offer no insights that might improve things for people suffering from mental illness, for neither appears to have any great faith in facts. Laing is a different matter. Whilst the excesses of his period as a counter-culture guru were self-indulgent, his early work on the meaning of the content of psychotic symptoms has eventually proven influential within psychiatry (Laing, 1960). Psychiatry can assimilate valid criticisms and new thinking within a strong conceptual framework and a clear set of ethical standards. Individual practitioners may sometimes betray these ideas and rules, but there is clarity as to what they are. Our belief in the strength of mainstream psychiatry rests on this. We reject the remaking of the profession and the creation of a post-modern psychiatry, because in such a remade world the rules would be uncertain and service users would have even fewer safeguards against charlatans than they have now.

Gramsci wrote of optimism of the will and pessimism of the intellect. By this he meant that to change the world, you need a determined belief that positive change is possible, tempered by a realistic understanding of the obstructions along the way. These ideas have an obvious relevance to psychiatry. The development of mental health services over the past twenty-five years has travelled down some blind alleys and has been marked by all manner of setbacks. Nonetheless, there has been substantial progress, especially in our alliance with patients. We have no doubt the experience of psychiatrists over the next twenty-five years will be similar. It will be, we believe, a worthwhile but challenging journey.

References

Anonymous (1981). The new psychiatry. *British Medical Journal*, **283**, 513–514.

Anonymous (1998). News: Mental Health Law to be tightened. *British Medical Journal*, **317**, 365.

Beardon, P.H.G., McGilchrist, M.M., McKendrick, A., McDevitt, D.G. and MacDonald, T.M. (1993). Primary non-compliance with prescribed medication in primary care. *British Medical Journal*, **307**, 846–848.

Bloch, S. and Reddaway, P. (1977). *Psychiatric Terror: How Soviet Psychiatry is Used to Suppress Dissent*. New York: Basic Books.

Briscoe, J., McCabe, R., Priebe, S. and Kallert, T. (2004). A national survey of psychiatric day hospitals. *British Journal of Psychiatry*, **28**, 160–163.

Burns, T., Catty, J., Dash, M., Roberts, C., Lockwood, A. and Marshall, M. (2007). Use of intensive case management to reduce time in hospital in people with severe mental illness: systematic review and meta-regression. *British Medical Journal*, **335**, 336. doi: 10.1136/bmj.39251.599259.55.

Burns, T., Knapp, M., Catty, J., Healy, A., Henderson, J., Watt, H. and Wright, C. (2001). Home treatment for mental health problems: a systematic review. *Health Technology Assessment*, **5**, 1–139.

Burns, T. and Priebe, S. (1999). Mental health care failure in England: myth and reality. *British Journal of Psychiatry*, **174**, 191–192.

Cohen, L.S., Friedman, J.M., Jefferson, J.W., Johnson, E.M. and Weiner, M.L. (1994). A re-evaluation of risk of in utero exposure to lithium. *Journal of the American Medical Association*, **271**, 2, 146–150.

Cramer, J.A. and Rosenheck, R. (1998). Compliance with medication regimens for mental and physical disorders. *Psychiatric Services*, **49**, 196–201.

Dawkins, R. (1987). *The Selfish Gene*, 2nd edn. Oxford: Oxford University Press.

Day, J.C., Bentall, R.P., Roberts, C., Randall, F., Rogers, A., Cattell, D., Healy, D., Rae, P. and Power, C. (2005). Attitudes towards antipsychotic medication: the impact of clinical variables and relationships with health professionals. *Archives of General Psychiatry*, **62**, 717–724.

Dean, C., Phillips, J., Gadd, E.M., Joseph, M. and England, S. (1993). Comparison of community based service with hospital based service for people with acute severe psychiatric illness. *British Medical Journal*, **307**, 473–476.

Department of Health (1990). The Care Programme Approach for people with mental illness. Joint Health/Social Services Circular HC(90) 23/LASS(90)II. London: Department of Health.

Department of Health (2005). *New ways of working for psychiatrists: Enhancing effective person-centred services*. London: Department of Health.

Ernst, E. (2002). Adulteration of Chinese herbal medicines with synthetic drugs: a systematic review. *Journal of Internal Medicine*, **252**, 2, 107–113.

Ferrier, I.N., MacMillan, I.C. and Young, A.H. (2001). The search for the wandering thymostat: a review of some developments in bipolar disorder research. *British Journal of Psychiatry*, **178**, 103–106.

Freeman, H. (2005). Psychiatry and the state in Britain. In *Psychiatric Cultures Compared*, eds. M. Gijswijt-Hofstra, H. Oosterhuis, J. Vijselaar and H. Freeman. Amsterdam: Amsterdam University Press.

Geddes, J.R., Burgess, S., Hawton, K., Jamison, K. and Goodwin, G.M. (2004). Long-term lithium therapy for bipolar disorder: systematic review and meta-analysis of randomised controlled trials. *American Journal of Psychiatry*, **161**, 217–222.

General Medical Council (2006). *Good Medical Practice*. London: GMC.

Glover, G., Arts, G. and Babu, K. S. (2006). Crisis resolution/home treatment teams and psychiatric admission rates in England. *British Journal of Psychiatry*, **189**, 441–445.

Gray, R., Leese, M., Bindman, J., Becker, T., Burti, L, David, A., Gournay, K., Kikkert, M., Koeter, M., Puschner, B., Schene, A., Thornicroft, G. and Tansella, M. (2006). Adherence therapy for people with schizophrenia. *British Journal of Psychiatry*, **189**, 508–514.

Hawkins, J.M., Archer, K.J., Stratowski, S.M. and Keck, P.E. (1995). Somatic treatment of catatonia. *International Journal of Psychiatry in Medicine*, **25**, 4, 345–369.

Kane, J.M., Eerdekens, M., Lindenmayer, J.P., Keith, S.J., Lesem, M. and Karcher, K. (2003). Long-acting injectable risperidone: efficacy and safety of the first long-acting atypical antipsychotic. *American Journal of Psychiatry*, **160**, 1125–1132.

Kenardy, J. (2000). The current status of psychological debriefing. *British Medical Journal*, **321**, 1032–1033.

Keown, P., Holloway, F. and Kuipers, E. (2002). The prevalence of personality disorders, psychotic disorders and the affective disorders amongst the patients seen by a community mental health team in London. *Social Psychiatry and Psychiatric Epidemiology*, **37**, 2, 225–229.

Killaspy, H. (2007). Assertive community treatment in psychiatry. *British Medical Journal*, **335**, 311–312.

Killaspy, H., Bebbington, P., Blizard, R., Johnson, S., Nolan, F., Pilling, S. and King, M. (2006). The REACT study: randomised evaluation of assertive community treatment in north London. *British Medical Journal*, **332**, 815–820.

Laing, R.D. (1960). *The Divided Self*. London: Tavistock Publications.

Leff, J., Trieman, N., Knapps, M. and Hallam, A. (2000). The TAPS project: a report of 13 years of research, 1985–1998. *Psychiatric Bulletin*, **24**, 165–168.

Lifton, R.J. (1986). *The Nazi Doctors: Medical Killing and the Psychology of Genocide*. New York: Basic Books.

Mental Health Policy Implementation Guide (2002). *Dual Diagnosis Good Practice Guide*. London: Department of Health.

McCabe, R., Heath, C., Burns, T. and Priebe, S. (2002). Engagement of patients with psychosis in the consultation: conversation analytic study. *British Medical Journal*, **325**, 1148–1151.

McCabe, R. and Priebe, S. (2004). The therapeutic relationship in the treatment of severe mental illness. *International Journal of Social Psychiatry*, **50**, 115–128.

McCreadie, R.G. (2002). Use of drugs, alcohol and tobacco by people with schizophrenia: case-control study. *British Journal of Psychiatry*, **181**, 321–325.

Monro, E. and Rumgay, J. (2000). Role of risk assessment in reducing homicides by people with mental illness. *British Journal of Psychiatry*, **176**, 116–120.

National Institute for Clinical Excellence (2002). Schizophrenia: core interventions in the treatment and management of schizophrenia. London: NICE.

Norfolk, Suffolk and Cambridgeshire Strategic Health Authority (2003). Independent inquiry into the death of David Bennett. Norfolk, Suffolk and Cambridgeshire Strategic Health Authority.

Parkman, S., Davies, S., Leese, M., Phelan, M. and Thornicroft, G. (1997). Ethnic differences in satisfaction with mental health services among representative people with psychosis in south London. *British Journal of Psychiatry*, **171**, 260–264.

Perkins, R. (2001). What constitutes success? The relative priority of service users' and clinicians' views of mental health services. *British Journal of Psychiatry*, **179**, 9–10.

Pilling, S., Bebbington, P., Kuipers, E., Garety, P., Geddes, J., Orbach, G. and Morgan, C. (2002). Psychological treatments in schizophrenia. I. Meta-analysis of family intervention and cognitive behavioural therapy. *Psychological Medicine*, **32**, 763–782.

Poole, R. and Brabbins, C. (1996). Drug induced psychosis. *British Journal of Psychiatry*, **168**, 135–138.

Poole, R. and Higgo, R. (2006). *Psychiatric Interviewing and Assessment*. Cambridge: Cambridge University Press.

Poole, R., Ryan, T. and Pearsall, A. (2002). The NHS, the private sector, and the virtual asylum. *British Medical Journal*, **325**, 349–350.

Priebe, S., Jones, G., McCabe, R., Briscoe, J. and Wright, D. (2006). Effectiveness and costs of acute day hospital treatment compared with conventional in-patient care. *British Journal of Psychiatry*, **188**, 243–249.

Priebe, S., Watts, J., Chase, M. and Matanov, A. (2005). Processes of disengagement and engagement in assertive outreach patients: qualitative study. *British Journal of Psychiatry*, **187**, 438–443.

Roberts, G. and Wolfson, P. (2004). The rediscovery of recovery: open to all. *Advances in Psychiatric Treatment*, **10**, 37–48.

Ryan, T., Hatfield, B., Sharma, I., Simpson, V. and McIntyre, A. (2007). A census study on independent mental health sector usage across seven strategic health authorities. *Journal of Mental Health*, **16**, 2, 243–253.

Scull, A. (1991). *The Asylum as Utopia: W.A.F Browne and the Mid-Nineteenth Century Consolidation of Psychiatry*. London: Routledge.

Stein, L.I. and Test, M.A. (1980). Alternatives to mental hospital treatment. *Archives of General Psychiatry*, **37**, 392–397.

Summerfield, D. (2004). Cross cultural perspectives on the medicalisation of human suffering. In *Post-Traumatic Stress Disorder. Issues and Controversies*, ed. G. Rosen. London: John Wiley.

Taylor, D., Paton, C. and Kerwin, R. (2007). *The Maudsley Prescribing Guidelines*, 9th edn. London: Informa Healthcare.

Thornicroft, G. and Susser, E. (2001). Evidence-based psychotherapeutic interventions in the community care of schizophrenia. *British Journal of Psychiatry*, **178**, 2–4.

Tudor Hart, J. (1971). The inverse care law. *Lancet*, **1**, 405–412.

Tungaraza, T. and Poole, R. (2007). Influence of drug company authorship and sponsorship on drug trial outcomes. *British Journal of Psychiatry*, **191**, 82–83.

Viguera, A.C., Nonacs, R., Cohen, L.S., Tondo, L., Murray, A. and Baldessarini, R.J. (2000). Risk of recurrence of bipolar disorder in pregnant and nonpregnant women after discontinuing lithium maintenance. *American Journal of Psychiatry*, **157**, 179–184.

Volz, A., Khorsand, V., Gillies, D. and Leucht, S. (2007). Benzodiazepines for schizophrenia. *Cochrane Database of Systematic Reviews*, 2007, Issue 1.

Wing, J.K. and Brown, G. (1970). *Institutionalism and Schizophrenia.* Cambridge: Cambridge University Press.

Yonkers, K.A., Wisner, K.L., Stowe, Z., Leibenluft, E., Cohen, L., Miller, L., Manber, R., Viguera, A., Suppes, T. and Altshuler, L. (2004). Management of bipolar disorder during pregnancy and the postpartum period. *American Journal of Psychiatry*, **161**, 608–620.

Index

abstinence, 153
abuse, 157–158
accountability, 161, 195–196
acute behavioural disturbances, 162–164, 167
adaptability, 19–20, 39, 64, 203–208, 211
addiction. *See* dependency; substance misuse
ADHD. *See* attention deficit hyperactivity disorder (ADHD)
adherence. *See* compliance and concordance
adherence therapy, 131
admissions, 70, 73–74, 77–79, 173, 186, 197–198
alcohol. *See* substance misuse
algorithms, prescribing, 140–143, 206–207
alternative therapies, 106–107
amitriptyline, 140–142
amphetamines, 168
anorexia nervosa, 102–103, 158–159
anti-therapeutic factors, 136
    see also substance misuse
anxiety
    in mental health professionals, 59, 62–63
    in patients, 19, 26, 39, 79, 93, 138–139, 146
assertive outreach teams (AOTs), 116, 132
assessments
    of contextual factors, 70
    for inpatient care, 70, 197–198
    of parenting skills, 155–157
    for treatment, 26–28, 31–32, 59–60, 156
    see also risk assessment
asylums. *See* institutions
attachment, mother–infant, 156–157
attention deficit hyperactivity disorder
    (ADHD), 208
autonomy
    in models of care, 98–99, 104, 194–195
    nurses and, 56, 65
    of patients, 68–69, 81, 85, 180, 198–200
    as treatment objective, 25, 176–177, 187
    see also mental capacity
away-days, 64

behavioural disturbances, 162–164, 167
behavioural family therapy, 180–181

benzodiazepines, 19, 146, 152, 166–167, 198
bipolar affective disorder
    management of, 130–131, 177–180
    substance misuse and, 28, 57, 114, 149–150
birth defects, 154
Boateng, Paul, 124
bonding, mother–infant, 156–157
boundaries
    in engagement, 11–12, 118, 185
    between teams, 46–47, 61
burn out, 204–205

cannabis. *See* substance misuse
carbamazepine, 144
care coordinators. *See* key workers
care programme model, 97–100, 103, 195
case loads, 50
    see also referrals
case notes, 40–41, 114, 135, 157–159, 162
case studies, 16
caution, excessive, 17–18, 161, 174
CBT. *See* cognitive behaviour therapy (CBT)
change
    in clinical practice, 64, 203–204
    patients and, 209
    psychiatrists and, 203–206, 208, 211
    in psychiatry, 7–8, 192–193, 208, 213–214
child protection services, 62–63, 155–156,
    170–171
children
    of patients, 65–66, 155–157, 170–171
    sex abuse in, 157–158
    treatment of, 197–198
chlorpromazine, 167
chronic fatigue syndrome, 208
chronic hallucinosis, 151–152
clinical dilemmas
    death penalty cases, 193–194
    difficult families, 196–197, 199
    idiosyncratic practice, 192–193
    inpatient admissions, 197–198
    late disclosure, 157–159
    overview, 149–150, 159–160, 191–192, 202

clinical dilemmas (*cont.*)
  patient choices, 198–200
  pregnancy and puerperium, 154–157
  substance misuse, 150–154
  treating colleagues, 200–201
  treatment without clear benefit, 201–202
  see also ethics
clinical hypotheses, 11
clinical practice
  burn out in, 204–205
  change in, 64, 203–204
  emergent disorders and, 208
  experience and, 16–18, 58–59
  innovation and, 7–8, 192–193, 208, 213–214
  new approaches to, 7–8, 206–208
  and scientific evidence, 13–16, 18
  skills required, 9–12
  see also clinical dilemmas; engagement
clinical skepticism, 10–11
clinicians. *See* psychiatrists
clouding of consciousness, 152
clozapine, 127–128, 138–139, 144
CMHTs. *See* Community Mental Health Teams
  (CMHTs)
cognitive behaviour therapy (CBT), 131,
  140–142, 180–181
cognitive impairments, 28, 102–103, 197–198
collaboration. *See* consultation and
  collaboration
commodity, health care as, 195
communication
  and engagement, 33–36, 78, 113–115,
    126–127, 135, 172
  during inpatient care, 165–166
  with patient families, 35
  among team members, 45–47, 58
  between teams, 54–55, 60–63
  terminology and, 34–35, 209–211
  treatment records, 40–41, 62–63, 114, 135,
    157–159, 162, 173
Community Mental Health Teams (CMHTs)
  advantages and disadvantages of, 53–54
  composition of, 46
  and inpatient care, 75–76, 82–85
  and outpatient clinics, 88–91
  referrals and, 59–61, 83–84
community psychiatry. *See* models of care;
  team work; treatment teams
complementary therapies, 106–107
complex problems
  late disclosure, 157–159
  overview, 149–150, 159–160
  pregnancy and puerperium, 154–157
  substance misuse, 150–154

compliance and concordance
  adherence therapy, 131
  depot antipsychotic medications and,
    129–130
  engagement and, 125–126, 132
  interventions for, 131–132
  non-compliance, 122–125
  overview, 121–122, 133
  reasons for, 125–126
  self-management strategies, 130–131
  side effects and, 126–129
compulsion/compulsory treatment. *See* legal
  compulsion
concordance. *See* compliance and
  concordance
confidentiality, 95
conflicts of interest, 15–16
consultation and collaboration, 54–55, 58–59,
    61, 174
  see also team work
contextual factors
  assessments and, 70
  complications of treatment, 149–150, 179
  defined, 10, 18–19, 148
  environmental, 71–73, 86, 138–139, 165
  and inpatient care, 79
  personality problems, 28, 182–184, 186
  situational, 163
  substance misuse, 150–154
  see also complex problems
contradictory observations, 17–18
control, 68–69, 93
  see also legal compulsion; physical restraint
coping vs mental health treatment, 26–28,
    38–39, 99
cost–benefit evaluations, 22–23
  see also clinical dilemmas; risk assessment
credibility, 113–115

day hospitals, 93–94
death, of patients, 170–171, 173–174
death penalty cases, 193–194
defensive practice, 173
delirium, 152
delirium tremens (DTs), 152
dependency
  on prescription medications, 19, 138–139,
    146, 152
  on professional care, 25–26, 32–33, 176–177
  as result of inpatient care, 69, 79, 82, 93,
    209
  see also substance misuse
depot antipsychotic medications, 129–130,
  187–188

depression
    medical tests for, 7
    post-intoxication, 152–153
    suicide risk and, 170–171, 183–184
    treatment of, 31–34, 140–141, 144
detention, long term, 82–85
developmental problems, 28, 102–103,
        197–198
diagnosis, 135, 149–150, 167–168, 209
discharge
    to consultant, 63
    planning for, 72–74, 176–177
disclosure, late, 157–159
disease model, of mental illness, 176
doctor–patient relationships. *See* engagement
doctors. *See* general practitioners (GPs);
        psychiatrists
dosage regimes
    changes in, 128, 142–143
    examples of, 140–141
    new medications and, 206–207
    prescribing algorithms, 142–143
    variable, 179–180
double blind studies, 15–16
drug interactions, 166–167
drug trials, 15–16
drug-induced psychosis, 151–153
drug-induced relapse, 152
DTs. *See* delirium tremens (DTs)
dual diagnosis, 149–150, 153–154

eating disorders, 158–159
ecstasy, 152, 168
    see also substance misuse
electroconvulsive treatment, 140–141, 143–146
emergent disorders, 208
emotional problems vs mental illness, 27–28,
        38, 99
empathy, 26
engagement
    adherence and, 125–126, 132
    boundaries in, 11–12, 118, 185
    challenges in, 19, 57, 114, 162, 202
    and change, 209
    communication and, 33–36, 78, 113–115,
        126–127, 135, 172
    difference and, 115–118, 198–200
    ethics of, 19, 112
    failure of, 112
    and forensic psychiatry, 193–194
    overview, 10, 97, 111, 120
    respect and dignity in, 118–120
    with suicidal patients, 169–173
    and team work, 116–117, 181–182

environmental factors, 71–73, 86, 138–139,
        165
ethics
    and accountability, 195–196
    in engagement, 19, 112
    and government policies, 193–195
    of informed consent, 194–195
    and legal compulsion, 24, 81–84
    and pharmaceutical companies, 206–207
    and reporting of abuse, 158
    and suicidal patients, 169
    and team work, 61
    in unusual settings, 95
euphemisms, 34–35, 209–211
excessive caution, 17–18, 161, 174
exclusion criteria, 59–60
external agencies, 59–63, 155–156

facilitation, 59, 63–64
failure of treatment, 38, 137, 146–147,
        201–202
family
    behavioural therapy, 180–182
    children of patients, 65–66, 155–157,
        170–171
    involvement in treatment, 35, 123, 158, 174,
        196–197, 199
flexibility, 19 20, 39, 64, 203 208, 211
fluclopenthixol, 166
fluoxetine, 32, 140–142
forcible injections, 166
forensic psychiatry, 193–194

gender issues, 118
general practitioners (GPs), 58–61
generalisations, risks of, 17–18
generic vs specialist teams, 52–54
"getting alongside" patients, 10
    see also engagement
"getting stuck". *See* treatment resistance
government policies, 21, 193–195
GPs. *See* general practitioners (GPs)

habilitation, 24
    see also rehabilitation
hallucinations, 151–152
haloperidol, 166
handicaps, secondary, 8, 18, 71, 86, 168
harm reduction, 153
Hart, Tudor, 98–99
Henderson Hospital, 70–71
Hillsborough disaster, 26–27
hospitalisation. *See* inpatient care
hypotheses, clinical, 11

inadequate treatment, 136
incapacity, mental, 100–104
incremental leave, 74
infants, 155–157
informed consent, 194–195
inpatient care
    and acute behavioural disturbances,
        163–167
    admissions, 73–74, 77–79, 186
    assessments for, 70, 197–198
    and community psychiatry, 68, 72–77
    control and restraint during, 68–69, 85, 165
    dependency and, 79, 82, 93
    environmental factors in, 8, 70–73, 86, 168
    intensive treatment, 70–71
    mothers and, 156–157
    nurses and, 73
    overview, 80
    of prisoners and the homeless, 94–95,
        105–106
    "rising acuity" in, 210
    of suicidal patients, 173
insight, of patients, 103–104, 125, 130–131
institutions, 8, 69, 71–73
    see also legal compulsion
interventions. See treatment
interviews, joint, 58
intolerance to medications, 127, 136
intoxication. See substance misuse
inverse care law, 98–99

joint interviews, 58
joint working, 56–58, 64, 153
    see also parallel working
Jones, Maxwell, 70–71
judicial killing, 193–194

key workers, 60–61, 74, 76–77, 92, 116, 200

late disclosure, 157–159
leadership, 50–51, 63–64, 204–205
legal compulsion
    appropriateness of, 81–84, 86–87, 104, 198
    justifications for, 24, 85, 164, 170–171
    and long-term detention, 82–85
    overview, 87
    psychiatric intensive care units, 86
    and therapeutic relationships, 191–192
    see also mental capacity; physical restraints
liability, 64–65, 161, 173
lifestyle, 115–116, 150
Lifton, Robert (*The Nazi Doctors*), 193
lithium carbonate, 140–141, 143, 154, 178–179
Liverpool Football Club, 1989 incident,
    26–27

long-term detention, 82–85
lorazepam, 138–139

MAOIs, 146
MAPPAs. *See* Multi-Agency Public Protection
    Arrangements (MAPPAs)
MCA. *See* Mental Capacity Act (MCA)
McNaughton, Daniel, 104–105
MDMA, 152, 168
    see also substance misuse
medical ethics. *See* ethics
medical paternalism, 49, 103, 194–195, 209
medical tests, for mental illness, 7–8
medications
    for acute behavioural disturbances,
        166–167
    dependency, 19, 138–139, 146
    discontinuation of, 147, 180
    intolerance to, 127, 136
    misuse of, 152
    new, 7–8, 206–208
    and patient control, 18, 85
    pharmacists' roles, 132
    pharmacokinetic stability, 128
    polypharmacy, 33, 39, 143
    side effects, 38–39, 126–129, 154–155, 178
    testing of, 15–16
    see also dosage regimes
meetings, 50, 62–63, 92
    see also ward rounds
mental capacity, 100–104
Mental Capacity Act (MCA), 101–102
mirtazapine, 142
models of care
    autonomy in, 98–99, 104, 194–195
    care programme vs patient-as-consumer
        model, 97–100, 103, 195
    cognitive behaviour vs behavioural family
        therapy, 180–182
    and criminal offenders, 104–106
    engagement and, 97
    holistic care, 106–107
    insight and responsibility, 103–104
    mental capacity and, 100–102
    overview, 107–108
    therapeutic community movement, 70–71
    see also inpatient care
monoamine oxidase inhibitors (MAOIs), 146
mood stabilisers. *See* lithium carbonate
Multi-Agency Public Protection Arrangements
    (MAPPAs), 62–63

National Health Service (NHS), 71, 79
Nazi Doctors, The (Lifton), 193
neologisms, 209–211

NHS. *See* National Health Service (NHS)
non-compliance, 122–125
non-pharmacological treatments, 207–208
no-return referrals, 146–147
normalcy, 123
nosology, 136–137, 208
nurses
   autonomy and, 56, 65
   engagement and, 57, 116
   and inpatient care, 73

objectives of treatment
   autonomy as, 25, 176–177, 187
   communication of, 35–36
   overview, 10, 29
   patient involvement in, 21–24
   and purpose of treatment, 21–24
   quality of life as, 21–24, 123, 147, 201
   rehabilitation and recovery as, 24–26
   and treatment resistance, 135, 185
objectivity, 11, 14–19, 205–206
olanzapine, 128, 140–141
onset of mental illness, 156
optimism, 39–40
orthodox vs complementary therapies,
   106–107
outpatient clinics, 88–92
overextended inpatient admissions, 70–79

PACT. *See* Psychiatric Assertive Community
   Treatment (PACT)
panic attacks, 153
paraldehyde, 168
parallel working, 56–57
   see also joint working
parenting skills, 155–157
partial hospitalisation, 93–94
   see also day hospitals
paternalism, 49, 103, 194–195, 209
pathoplastic reactions, 151
patient choice. *See* patient-as-consumer
   model
patient-as-consumer model, 97–100, 103, 195
patients
   autonomy of, 68–69, 81, 85, 180, 198–200
   behaviour of, 119–120, 198–200
   change and, 209
   children of, 65–66, 155–157
   death of, 170–171, 173–174
   and emergent disorders, 208
   expectations of, 26, 34, 39–40, 74, 99–100,
     145–146
   family involvement, 35, 123, 158, 174,
     196–197, 199
   histories, 40–41, 114, 135, 157–159, 162

   insight of, 103–104, 125, 130–131
   involvement in treatment, 21–24, 34–35, 202
   mental capacity of, 100–103
   quality of life of, 21–24, 123, 147, 201
   responsibility for actions, 103–106, 176–177
   see also engagement; substance misuse;
     wellness
pediatrics. *See* children
perinatal treatment, 154–155
personality problems, 28, 182–184, 186
pharmaceutical companies, 15–16, 206–207
pharmacists, 132
pharmacokinetic stability, 128
physical restraints, 18, 85, 165
   see also control; legal compulsion
physicians. *See* general practitioners (GPs);
   psychiatrists
PICUs. *See* psychiatric intensive care units
   (PICUs)
plans for treatment, 36–37, 60–61, 78–79
police
   and acute behavioural disturbances, 163,
     168
   interface with, 22–23, 62–63, 83–84
   and zero tolerance policies, 119–120
policies, government. *See* government policies
polypharmacy, 33, 39, 143
practitioners. *See* general practitioners (GPs);
   nurses; psychiatrists
pre-birth meetings, 155–156
pregnancy, 154–155
prescribing algorithms, 140–143, 206–207
Priebe, Stefan, 132
prioritising of treatment, 32, 36–37, 39
prisoners, 94–95, 105–106, 193–194
probability, 15
process, 10
Psychiatric Assertive Community Treatment
   (PACT), 116
psychiatric intensive care units (PICUs), 86
psychiatrists
   and change, 203–206, 208, 211
   and legal compulsion, 86–87
   and patient deaths, 170–171, 173–174
   responsibilities of, 64–65, 86–87, 119
   and scientific evidence, 13, 16, 18–19
   suicide risk among, 200–201
   and team effectiveness, 47–51, 58–59, 64–65
   see also clinical practice; engagement; ethics
psychiatry
   change in, 7–8, 192–193, 208, 213–214
   vs psychology, 214–215
   scientific models and, 13, 18–19, 214
   technical innovations and, 7–8, 192–193,
     208

psychoanalysis, 192–193
psychology vs psychiatry, 214–215
psychotic symptoms from substance misuse, 151–153
public safety, 62–63, 85, 158
puerperium, 155–157

qualitative studies, 16
quality of life, 21–24, 201
quantitative studies, 15–16
quetiapine, 129

race, 86, 117–118, 198–200
Randomised Controlled Trials (RCTs), 15–16
rapid readmission, 79
rapport. *See* engagement
RCTs. *See* Randomised Controlled Trials (RCTs)
reactive treatment, 30–34, 37
record keeping, 40–41, 62–63, 114, 135, 157–159, 162, 173
recovery, 25–26, 39–40, 176–177, 186–188
see also wellness
Recovery Model, 25–26
referrals, 50, 59–61, 146–147, 156
refractory disorders. *See* treatment resistance
rehabilitation, 24–25, 71
see also wellness
relapse signatures, 130–131
relapses, 152, 155
religion and spirituality, 107
resistance, to treatment. *See* treatment resistance
respiratory depression, 167
restraints. *See* physical restraints
retreats, 64
"rising acuity", 210
risk assessments
generalisations and, 17–18
for mental illness, 105
and patient communication, 34–35, 37
of polypharmacy, 33, 39, 143
of prescription medications, 19, 38–39, 126–129, 152, 154–155, 178
of relapse, 152, 155
of suicide, 74
and teams, 65–66
risk management
and acute behavioural disturbances, 162–164, 167–168
overview, 161–162, 174–175
with psychosocial interventions, 180–182
and suicidal patients, 168–171, 173
risk-averse practice, 17–18, 161, 174

safety, public, 62–63, 85, 158
schizophrenia
management of, 28, 138–139, 177–180, 187–188
secondary handicaps and, 71
stereotypes and, 117–118
substance misuse and, 105–106, 149–154, 199
see also depot antipsychotic medications
scientific evidence
and clinical experience, 13–16, 18
and complementary therapies, 106–107
and new medications, 207
relevance of, 15
and treatment resistance, 134, 142
scientific models, 13, 18–19, 214
second opinions, 54–55, 101, 144–145
secondary handicaps, 8, 18, 71, 86, 168
security, 62–63, 85, 158
self-awareness, 11
Serbsky Institute, 193
setbacks, 33, 37–39
sexual abuse, 157–158
shared understanding, 34–36
side effects, 38–39, 126–129, 154–155, 178
situational factors, 163
skepticism, clinical, 10–11
social workers. *See* key workers; key workers
sodium amytal, 168
specialist vs generic teams, 52–54
spirituality and religion, 107
standards of evidence, 16
statistical evidence, 15
stereotypes, 86, 117–118, 198–200
stigma, 122–123
strategic treatment
communication and, 34–36, 40–41
overview, 41
vs reactive treatment, 30–34
sequencing of, 36–37
setbacks in, 37–39
"stuckness". *See* treatment resistance
subcultures, 94, 115–116, 150
subjectivity, 17–18
substance misuse
and acute behavioural disturbances, 163, 168
as complicating factor, 28, 135–136, 138–139, 150–154, 199
dual diagnosis, 149–150, 153–154
harm reduction vs abstinence, 153
and legal compulsion, 84
and patient responsibility, 104
of prescription medications, 152

psychotic symptoms from, 151–153
and timing of treatment, 32, 36–37, 39
and treatment settings, 72
suicide
  patient death from, 170–171, 173–174
  risk of, 34–35, 74, 168–173, 200–201
symptom abatement, 146–147, 187

team work
  consultation and collaboration, 54–55,
    58–59, 61, 174
  engagement and, 57, 112
  with external agencies, 59–63
  joint working, 56–58, 64, 153
  member dynamics, 45–46, 56, 63–66
  overview, 67
  transfers of care, 62–63, 74
  see also treatment teams
teams. See treatment teams
technical innovations, 7–8, 192–193, 208,
    213–214
technical terminology, 34–35, 209–211
television, 182
teratogenic risk, 154
termination of treatment, 40
  see also recovery; rehabilitation; wellness
theory of mind, 103–104
therapeutic community movement, 70–71
therapeutic relationships. See engagement
Three Hospitals Study, 18, 71
time, perception of, 203
timing of treatment, 32, 36–37, 39, 158
TMS. See transcranial magnetic stimulation
    (TMS)
tolerance, for mentally ill, 21, 25, 85–87,
    122–123
trajectory of improvement, 11, 38, 40
transcranial magnetic stimulation (TMS),
    144
transference, 118
transfers of care, 62, 74
treatment
  assessments for, 26–28, 31–32, 59–60, 156
  beneficiaries of, 22–23, 26–29, 201–202
  vs coping, 26–28, 38–39, 99
  criteria for, 26–28, 59–61, 77–79, 99–100,
    105–106
  delivery of, 8–9
  duration of, 148, 167, 176–177
  failure of, 38, 137, 146–147, 201–202
  inadequate, 136
  with new medications, 206–208
  non-pharmacological, 207–208
  patient involvement in, 21–24, 34–35, 202

personality problems and, 185–186
plans, 36–37, 60–61, 78–79
prioritisation of, 32, 36–37, 39, 158
purpose of, 21–24
reactive, 30–34, 37
records of, 40–41, 62–63, 114, 135, 157–159,
    162, 173
refusal of, 198–200
setbacks in, 33, 37–39
by teams vs one-on-one, 47
termination of, 40
see also clinical dilemmas; medications;
    strategic treatment; treatment teams
treatment adherence rates, 124
treatment objectives
  autonomy as, 25, 176–177, 187
  communication of, 35–36
  overview, 10, 29
  patient involvement in, 21–24
  and purpose of treatment, 21–24
  quality of life as, 21–24, 123, 147, 201
  rehabilitation and recovery as, 24–26
  and treatment resistance, 135, 185
treatment resistance
  factors in, 134–135, 137
  overview, 134, 147–148
  prescribing algorithms and, 140–143
  vs treatment failure, 137, 140–141, 146–147
  types of, 137
  and unorthodox treatments, 138–139,
    144–146
  see also clinical dilemmas
treatment settings
  day hospitals, 93–94
  office based treatment, 91–92
  outpatient clinics, 88–92
  overview, 88, 95–96
  for prisoners and the homeless, 94–95,
    105–106
  see also inpatient care; institutions; models
    of care
treatment teams
  collaboration among, 54–55, 58–59, 61,
    174
  composition of, 45–47
  disruptive factors in, 49, 52, 116–117
  effectiveness of, 45–48, 51–52, 168
  engagement in, 116–117, 181–182
  generic vs specialist, 52–54
  and inpatient care, 72–73
  leadership of, 50–51, 63–64, 204–205
  management of, 47–50, 206
  and new treatments, 208
  and outpatient clinics, 92

treatment teams (*cont.*)
  overview, 55
  responsibility in, 149–150
  see also team work
triangle of forces
  balance of, 19–20, 208
  clinical experience, 16–18
  context, 18–19
  overview, 13–21
  scientific evidence, 14–16
Tudor Hart's inverse care law, 98–99

venlafaxine, 143

ward rounds, 75–77
wellness
  medication and, 177–180
  overview, 176–177, 188
  personality problems and, 182–184, 186
  see also recovery; rehabilitation
withdrawal states, 152

zero tolerance policies, 119–120